# CONQUERING CONFIDENCE

JAY GURDEN

# DEDICATION

This book is dedicated to everyone who has made the
resolution to tackle their impostor syndrome. Have no
doubt. You can do this!

# CONTENTS

Acknowledgments    i

Impostor Syndrome and Me    1

What is Impostor Syndrome?    5

Definitions of Impostor Syndrome    17

The Critical Inner Voice    33

Impostor Syndrome and the Canine World    36

Fear of Failure and the Stress Response    40

Signs of Impostor Syndrome    47

What Causes Impostor Syndrome?    54

Conquering the Inner Critic    57

Combatting Impostor Syndrome in Personality Types    61

Combatting Impostor Syndrome Outside of Personality Types    65

Cognitive Restructuring    83

Cognitive Behavioural Therapy    97

Self-Esteem and Self-Acceptance     125

Mindfulness     133

Final Thoughts     147

About the Author     149

# ACKNOWLEDGMENTS

This project has been made possible by the support of a small group of people. My family have been so, so supportive of my writing efforts, and I'm not sure I have the words to describe the support my husband Daniel gives me, in writing, and in life in general. This book came about as the result of an offhand comment to someone about whether she could please write me a course in how to deal with impostor syndrome. Her response was 'You could write one!' I may not have written a course, but I did rise to her challenge, and here is the concrete evidence. Sally, thank you for pushing me to do the things I don't realise I can do, and supporting me while I do them.

# IMPOSTOR SYNDROME AND ME

Hello. My name is Jay and I suffer from impostor syndrome. That is such a short sentence and yet it represents years of mental struggles, ups and downs, and many, many hours of frustration and tears. It was not an easy sentence to say to start with, but once I had recognised what was going on and could bring myself to admit that fact, I could start to find ways of managing and combatting it.

To describe the situation more accurately, I have undergone frequent struggles with impostor syndrome. When I look back at the various jobs I have held in a variety of industries, the signs have always been there. I did not realise what was occurring at the time but viewing those situations from a position of being several years older and maybe just a little bit wiser than I used to be, I can see it all too well.

Impostor syndrome is so pervasive that, for many years, I refused to believe others that told me I should speak up more and have more faith in my own abilities. My knowledge of the subject at hand was extensive and up to date, and my skillset varied and expansive enough to deal with anything that would come up from day to day on the farm with the livestock, although I could never make myself truly realise that and believe it. Every situation found me second guessing myself and looking for the person that really knew what they were doing, that knew how to deal with what was going on better than I ever could. I could never bring myself to acknowledge that in many of these situations, the person that actually knew best what to do and how to deal with the matter at hand was, in fact, me.

In all honesty, my impostor syndrome has been messing with me for pretty much my entire life, but it really came into its own and sank its teeth in when I released my first book, 'Fight or Fright? A Reactive Dog Guardian's Handbook' in early 2019. I had an initial period of looking at the live online book listing with the sense of utter excitement and joy, and again when I held a physical copy in my hands, this thing that I had created from a blank page up to a book. But then the thoughts started coming. Who on earth do you think you are to write a book? Nobody is ever going to want to read THAT thing! What makes you think you can be a writer anyway, especially about dogs? You know nothing about dogs, especially reactive ones. You haven't even managed to sort your own dog out yet.' (Side note: those of us that share our lives with the complex, special dogs that go under the label of 'reactive dogs' know that there is no 'sorting them out' or 'fixing them' in that way!)

In the impostor syndrome twisted part of my brain it did not matter about the fact that I wrote the book from the perspective of someone that did understand the subject matter very well, and wrote to help the people who were in the same position I had first been in with my own complicated canine. Never mind the hours and hours of study I had put in taking courses in many aspects of dogs, including training, general behaviour and reactive behaviour specialist courses among others. All the books, papers, articles, blogs and scientific papers I had tracked down and read. I put in an awful lot of hours working towards the idea of starting out on a career as a dog trainer. For various reasons that have no connection to impostor syndrome or to anything contained here the training career has not occurred, but that knowledge and the research skills studying has earned me have stood me in good stead developing my canine writing career.

Those damaging negative thoughts still nag at me with their so very sharp teeth sometimes. They have been very unimpressed through the entire process of writing this book and other associated projects I have undertaken concerning the same subject matter. I have spent the last few months fighting impostor syndrome about my impostor syndrome, my ability to deal with it, and why I could possibly think I could help others to understand. Looking back on the mental gymnastics of convincing myself I actually could write this book, I now find it almost funny in some ways. I refuse to listen to those thoughts any longer. They no longer get to have any power over me, they do not get to drain my mental energy and I do not give them time to influence my thoughts, feelings or behaviour.

By the time we reach the other end of this book, learning more along the way about what impostor syndrome is, how it holds us back, and some tools to combat its effects, hopefully you will begin to realise that they do not have to have that kind of power over you and your mind any more either.

# WHAT IS IMPOSTOR SYNDROME

• Tom Hanks – multiple award-winning actor
• Sheryl Sandberg- chief operating officer at Facebook
• David Bowie – multiple award-winning iconic singer and actor
• Serena Williams – most singles titles of any tennis player in the Open Era
• Tina Fey- award-winning comedian, actress, producer and writer
• Maya Angelou – Pulitzer Prize nominee and Grammy winning writer and poet
• Sonia Sotomayor - first Hispanic United States Supreme Court justice
• Neil Gaiman – multiple award-winning writer
• Neil Armstrong – first man on the moon

What do the people on the list above have in common?

This list of notable people holds some of the best-known names on our planet, and others who have broken through all kinds of barriers in the course of their lives. These in some cases legendary high achievers in their respective varied fields have all publicly admitted that they have struggled with the confidence sapping, mentally draining effects of Impostor Syndrome, that lingering, crippling fear that at any moment they will be revealed as frauds, incompetent and not worthy of the accolades they have earned. Many more names, equally well known, have also referred to their struggles with the phenomenon, showing just how widespread the problem is.

These feelings are, as mentioned above, relatively common but the name impostor syndrome is not widely known. A survey carried out in 2019 revealed that 85% of adults surveyed, all of whom had been established in their current roles for a minimum of 3 years, experienced feelings of inadequacy or incompetence at work, with 80% of men and 90% of women reporting them. Only 25% of those asked, however, had heard of the term impostor syndrome.

Of those reporting these intrusive thoughts regarding their performance, such as thinking their success came from luck or thinking praise they received underserved, 25% said these thoughts were with them often or all of the time. This demonstrates just how much capacity the impostor syndrome type of thinking has to cause us mental distress by damaging our self-esteem and causing us to have serious doubts about our abilities, knowledge, and skills.

Many of us experience, at least at some point, that terrible nagging feeling of doubt in ourselves and our abilities, skills, and talents. In the short term, when taking on a new job or just starting out on a new project, these thoughts and feelings are quite natural and understandable. If, once the job is more familiar or the project is completed, these feelings dissipate there is no problem. If they linger and worsen, leading to a constant state of self-doubt, and a possible lack of self-confidence, then this could mean they are symptoms of the uncomfortable mental well-being and career threatening experience that is impostor syndrome. A constant, wearying perceiving of ourselves as being fraudulent, faking our way into whatever success we have achieved. A sneaking idea that, behind the false façade of an adequate professional, is in fact an incompetent failure. If not tackled, impostor syndrome can become a self-fulfilling problem as our thoughts fall into a habitual pattern of claiming to ourselves that we are frauds, and not able to do some of the things involved in our careers competently and confidently.

Impostor syndrome is not one singular thing that we can define easily. The nature of our individuality means that every person who suffers with impostor syndrome has a slightly different experience of it. This complicates the issue a little further, as it can manifest in a number of slightly different ways, involving different ways of thinking. To describe it in the most inclusive way of the variety of experiences possible, impostor syndrome is a collection of thoughts and feelings that project feelings of inadequacy and/or intellectual fraudulence. The central idea projected is that the sufferer is not good at their job, but has managed, through luck or by fooling their peers, to convince those around them that they are competent professionals. Any success the sufferer has had cannot be accepted and internalised, but any errors or perceived failures can be dwelt on for far longer than is necessary or healthy, and projected outwards to others, deflecting and discounting the positive feedback that was earned in a valid way.

There are times in all of our lives, family, social, or work related, when a certain amount of worry and stress is to be expected. Any kind of transition in personal or professional lives is almost certainly going to create a period of uncertainty and potentially cause anxiety. Creating a new canine related business for example, or taking the step to move from making your living solely from dog walking to add home boarding, or beginning to work as a canine coach, or offering canine behavioural consultations, is a big step. In any of those changes, a certain amount of trepidation is to be expected. We all feel nervous at times. The difference is that, for those struggling with impostor syndrome, these thoughts can become all-consuming and do not dissipate with time. While a certain amount of worry about a transition is natural and understandable, it is important to think about just where this line sits, and where it starts to become a problem and bordering on unhealthy.

As stated earlier, impostor (also spelled imposter) syndrome is a commonly experienced but not necessarily widely known psychological phenomenon. It leads those suffering with it to experience chronic, potentially mentally crippling self-doubt amongst other damaging thoughts and beliefs. Sufferers will often view themselves as unintelligent, lacking ability and talent to meet the demands of their roles, that they are fooling others into believing them competent, and that their successes are down to luck or hard work. These feelings of fraudulence, incompetence, or inadequacy are pervasive and persistent and can create massive sensations of stress and anxiety, even against a history of accomplishments and successes that should, in theory, prove that the feelings are not based in truth.

Despite the word 'syndrome' in the commonly used name, impostor syndrome is not an actual psychological condition. It is a pattern of negative thoughts and emotions. A habitual thinking and feeling routine that the brain follows in certain situations connected to work and performance. A set of psychological barriers that prevent sufferers from internally accepting their successes and value in their professional lives. It is an experience, an inner belief that, because of the way we hold it within ourselves, and how it involves the very core of how we see ourselves, is very hard to tackle. Whether known as impostor syndrome, impostor phenomenon, the impostor experience, impostorism, or fraud syndrome, sufferers doubt their own level of knowledge and abilities, believing themselves inadequate and in constant danger of being 'found out' as not as clever or talented or worthwhile as others see them. They lack the ability to internally recognise and acknowledge their own worth and the way in which their skills, talents, and abilities make them a successful and worthwhile part of their professional world. Sufferers go through ha continual process of comparing them to others in their personal and professional lives, and will find themselves lacking in comparison, regardless of the truth of their equality. No matter the successes they have had, or the accomplishments they have acquired, these people will still see themselves as fakes, always on the verge of discovery. When discussing others, they will emphasise that person's strengths while talking down their own. Instead, they talk about their own skill and knowledge deficits and minimise those of others in their professional sphere.

Impostor syndrome causes the sufferer to lack the ability to accept praise, discounting any recognition and positive feedback they receive, or achievements and accomplishments they may attain. Negative feedback or anything that is in any way connected with their mistakes or failures, or that they can connect with their perceived deficits will be dwelt on for long periods, or even indefinitely, as the sufferer fixates on their flaws. As those suffering from impostor syndrome can struggle massively with fearing failure and the associated shame and humiliation, this adds into the negative psychological state, which makes the entire situation even worse.

Those struggling with impostor syndrome can find themselves procrastinating and putting off doing tasks, leaving them with a mountain of work to complete at the last minute in an attempt to get things done. This can lead to a kind of paralysis, an inability to be able to make progress against their fear of not being able to finish in time, or indeed to finish successfully at all. A certain kind of self-defence can come into play, where the sufferer might avoid challenging themselves and stretching their boundaries because of their fear of failure, or worries about being able to keep up the same level of work and ability. Because of the way in which they expect themselves to perform at the highest levels consistently and dwell on any perceived failure, they cannot permanently escape not reaching their own expectations and therefore will, at some point, experience disappointment with their performance and results.

Some of the patterns of thought and behaviour surrounding the issue of impostor syndrome are somewhat ritualistic in their nature, and become almost a superstition, with the allocation of a new task or project prompting a repetitive pattern of thinking, each time following the same path. As with anything concerning functions that take place in the brain, something that takes a particular path makes it easier for that path to be later followed again. Neurons are specialised cells in the nervous system that are designed to carry signals around the body. To use the most simple explanation, they carry information from all around the body to the brain, and then carry signals from the brain to the relevant body areas or organs to respond as that information requires. Once a pattern of movement of signals along the neurons has been established in the brain, called a neural pathway, it is likely that a similar situation in the future will result in the same neural pathway being followed. The more this happens, the more the patterns of thought, behaviour and action are repeated, the easier it becomes for that pathway to be followed, until the pathway becomes the default. Think of it as being something like a pathway across a field of grass. The more times feet travel over that same strip of grass, the clearer the path is marked out and the easier it becomes to follow.

One of the major difficulties of living with impostor syndrome is that the sufferer fears failure. Achieving success is not always an automatic antidote, however logical that may seem. For some, success may breed further anxiety, as it increases the pressure of maintaining performance at a certain level. The more they achieve at that level, the more they feel exposed and vulnerable. To avoid that feeling, they stop pushing further as a form of self-protection against what they see as inevitable discovery of their limitations. Fear can be a central element of impostor syndrome. Sufferers fear failure above all, but it can also extend to feeling fear around the concept of being evaluated in any way, of not being able to continue what success they have managed so far, and of being seen as less capable than others around them. The practice of limiting ourselves, avoiding new opportunities, potential new services that our businesses can offer and whole new areas of interest, can be massively damaging to personal and professional growth, and can seriously stunt career potential.

Living with impostor syndrome can be confidence sapping and mentally draining, leading to a life that may be filled with constant stress and anxiety, with all of the effects long term stress can have on mental and physical health. Feelings of concern, anxiety and fear can be frequently experienced, and depression could be a result of the constant struggle to maintain the image of success while feeling like a fraud, with the almost irresistible urge to look over a shoulder in anticipation of being outed as a fake. Impostor syndrome can have close effects with personal and personality factors. The connection with the concept of social anxiety is quite easy to see. Both involve difficulties in relating one's self-worth to others, and having problems accurately seeing how the sufferer fits in amongst their peers. In both cases, sufferers will not see themselves as belonging in their surroundings, socially or professionally. A history of anxiety or depression can leave a tendency to struggle with self-worth and self-esteem. This inability to value themselves and their talents pushes the sufferer towards the thoughts that they cannot be responsible for their successes, and that they must be due to luck, chance, being 'in the right place at the right time' or the effects of hard work. Any failure to attain their goals in just the way they would want is dwelt on and seen as a sign of their lack of worth, further damaging self-esteem.

Impostor syndrome is often seen to be linked with generalised feelings of low self-confidence and doubting oneself. Although there is an obvious overlap between impostor syndrome and issues around low self-esteem, anxiety, and depression, impostor syndrome is not tied to these, and seems to be very much its own separate issue.

Something that can be seen in many cases of

impostor syndrome is something called self-handicapping. This functions as both a method by which sufferers attempt to mitigate the effects of impostor syndrome on themselves and as a self-fulfilling part of the issue. As a cognitive tool, self-handicapping allows people to protect themselves from the idea of failing or not measuring up to the standards they want, and from the consequent issues with their self-esteem.

Self-handicapping is a common behaviour among humans and links with impostor syndrome in that it can cause people to avoid challenging themselves professionally and intellectually. Doing so provides a way to protect one's self-esteem as it reduces the likelihood of failure. Another method of self-handicapping involves creating obstacles, either real or theoretical, as an opportunity to 'explain away' failure if the self-sabotage is successful and failure does occur. This means that sufferers can externalise their failures and internalise their successes. While self-handicappers can accept praise and credit for some of their achievements, they are also providing themselves with ready excuses for their failures. One of the common methods of self-handicapping in impostor syndrome is procrastination, putting off tackling the task until the timescale for completion is almost unfeasibly short.

Since the first academic mention of the concept

of impostor syndrome, a number of different experts have expanded the thinking and theories around the subject, leading to a number of different names and definitions of what impostor syndrome is and how to define whether someone is suffering from it. Below are listed some of these different names and details of how they are each defined.

# DEFINITIONS OF IMPOSTOR SYNDROME

## Impostor Phenomenon

## Clance and Imes

The term impostor phenomenon was the first to be applied, coined in 1978, by the researchers Dr. Pauline Rose Clance and Dr. Suzanne Imes. They undertook a study involving more than 150 high achieving women, all of whom had received formal recognition of their professional excellence, and had achieved high standards of academic success, either by the earning of higher education qualifications such as degrees, or through the form of standardised testing scores. Despite this concrete objective evidence of their achievements in these ways, the women surveyed were not able to internally acknowledge their successes, instead explaining them as the result of external factors including luck, being in the 'right place at the right time' or others around them overestimating their intelligence and abilities.

Clance and Imes concluded that this lack of ability in many to own their successes came from a number of potential causes such as societal and cultural expectations, gender stereotypes and early family dynamics. They thought after this initial study that the impostor phenomenon was largely a female experience. Research that is more recent has discovered that gender does not appear to be as strong a contributing factor as first thought following those earliest studies, although those belonging to minorities in any area of experience or industry do seem to be more prone.

Clance discussed in a 1985 paper characteristics of the family unit and its function that may contribute towards the perpetuation of impostor phenomenon, as she terms it. These centre around the child's own perception of their intelligence and talents compared to other family members while they were growing up, how strongly prized intellectual ability is within the family unit, and the method and consistency with which praise is given or withheld for rewarding achievements. All of these affect how the growing child values achievements and the importance of various achievement types, which can follow through into their adult lives. It is still unclear exactly what causes impostor syndrome but studies have found a potential link between parents who are over-protective and have a greater degree of perceived control over their children. This, potentially also linked together with lower levels of self-esteem in the child, seem to predict a higher likelihood of impostor syndrome becoming a problem for an individual.

Dr. Clance laid out in 1985 a list of six dimensions that can aid in distinguishing the issue of impostor syndrome:

# 1) The impostor cycle

This is somewhat of a vicious cycle and in incredibly pervasive and persistent. The initial step is the arrival of a task that is achievement related. This can be in the form of a work assignment, an assessment for an educational course, or a new project for a business, as examples. Once the task has arrived on the horizon, it triggers feelings straight away such as anxiety about completing the task, worrying and experiencing feelings of self-doubt. Typically these worries will result in one of two reactions, either procrastination or over-preparing.

Procrastination allows the person to 'bury their head in the sand' for a while, but eventually there will be a huge effort to finish the job, accompanied by extra levels of frantic stress and worry. Once the task is completed, they may feel good about it for a while, enjoying a brief period of relief and sense of accomplishment. As this fades, however, the worry can then begin about the next task to come up. Any feedback they receive that carries a positive slant will receive immediate deflection and dismissal, and the success is put down to luck or chance, reducing its effects and influence on mental state.

If the reaction to the task is to over prepare, the same period of feeling they have accomplished something and relief at having completed the task will result, but the completion is attributed to having worked hard rather than their own level of ability, talent and knowledge. The sufferer claims that anyone who could work as hard could complete the task to the same level of proficiency.

In either case, the result is not seen as the consequence of true intelligence, ability or experience. Positive feedback is rejected and discounted, so does nothing towards personal recognition of their own successes, and does absolutely nothing to improve the situation when another task arises. This perpetuates the impostor cycle, leading to stronger feelings of fraudulence, anxiety and self-doubt. Because of the way that positive feedback is rejected, continued successes will also cause the feeling of fraudulence to increase in strength. The more fraudulent someone feels they are, the more they worry about being caught out or discovered, increasing anxiety levels, and making the cycle stronger than ever, as they are constantly fearing being 'exposed' at any moment.

Clance also observed that those suffering with the impostor phenomenon could become fixed on always working in the same way, believing that changing their style would result in failure.

## 2) A need to be the very best

Some battling with impostor syndrome feel a deep and urgent need to be the absolute very best in their field compared to their peers. If this is not the case, they may possibly dismiss the extent of their talents and believe that they are not intelligent or talented. It is not good enough for them to be very good or even excellent at what they do. Only the very pinnacle of the industry will do.

## 3) The super being

This dimension bears close links to the one above. These individuals hold a high expectation of themselves to be able to complete tasks in every single aspect of their lives without any flaws. This leads to the setting of standards that are almost unattainable, and they then experience massive disappointment, becoming overwhelmed and generalising themselves as utter failures when they cannot achieve these standards from the start, and achieve them consistently every single time.

## 4) Fear of failure

Tasks promote anxiety as the setting of something that requires achievement focuses the sufferer's mind straight away on the possibility of failure. Any chance of making a mistake or not performing at the very highest of standards may create feelings in the individual of humiliation and shame as they feel they then reveal themselves as not good enough for what they are doing, no matter how unfair this feeling may in fact be. A fear of failure is one of the most common factors in impostor syndrome. It can lead the sufferer to attempt to reduce their risk of failure by overworking, which then feeds back in to the impostor cycle, or to limit the scope of what they will attempt, as lessening the ambition of a task also lessens the chance of failure.

## 5) Denial of competence and discounting praise

Because sufferers cannot internally accept and acknowledge their successes, they are unable to accept praise and see it as a true and valid response to what they have done. Instead, they will show a tendency to push external factors as the reason the task was successfully completed. Further to that, sufferers may often actually go in search of evidence to 'prove' that they do not merit the praise and validation they receive. Others can view this as a display of false modesty and humility but this is not the case, as the sufferer genuinely believes they do not deserve the praise.

## 6) Fear and guilt about success

This factor links in with the concern around the perceived negative consequences of the sufferer's previous successes. This can connect back to early family dynamics as, if successes are perceived as unusual in the sufferer's family, they can begin to feel disconnected and growing more distant from their family as a result of being 'different' to the rest. The feeling of difference from their family (or colleagues in later life) can create a situation of feeling overwhelmed, and a fear of rejection because of these differences and that perception of disconnection from friends, colleagues, or loved ones.

This sensation of feeling overwhelmed by success also feeds in to the fear that greater success leads on to greater demands and expectations, making the situation increasingly more intense. Because the person concerned has worries about being able to maintain the level of performance already achieved the idea that more might be expected or requested, that more responsibility might be assigned, creates extra stress. It brings extra concern that they will be 'caught out', that their self-perceived intellectual fraudulence will be revealed.

To consider someone as struggling with impostor syndrome according to Dr. Clance's definition of it as impostor phenomenon, at least two of the above characteristics must be present. Dr. Clance developed a scale that allows people to assess how they compare to others in their possible experience of the phenomenon. It is available for personal use on her website.

* * * * *

## J.C. Harvey and C Katz

In 1985 these authors defined what we know as impostor syndrome, although they still titled it impostor phenomenon as Clance and Imes did previously, as a psychological effect, resulting in strong feelings of phoniness and fraudulence when an achievement related task arises, which feelings the sufferer will then struggle with in hiding. Their description of the syndrome involves three core factors.

1) A feeling of fraudulence, the belief that they have fooled others concerning the level of their knowledge, abilities and talents.

2) A fear of being exposed. As sufferers have convinced themselves that they are impostors, consequently they live in constant fear of being 'discovered' as fakes.

3) An inability to take ownership of their achievements and successes as a result of their internal qualities, including ability, intelligence or skills.

All three of these criteria must be present for their definition to be met, making it much more specific, but very familiar to those that do suffer with impostor syndrome as these feelings are the most commonly reported effects on sufferers.

* * * * *

# Neurotic Imposture

In a 2005 article M. Kets de Vries described the concept of impostor syndrome under the name 'neurotic imposture' and defined it as involving high achievers who believe they are really complete fakes, To an outside observer these people are highly – even remarkably – accomplished, but internally they view themselves subjectively as frauds. Neurotic imposture is a psychological phrase, which separates sufferers from the concept of false humility and deliberate playing down of abilities and achievements to appear humble and to be liked. Because of neurotic imposture, a great many very talented and able people are unable to enjoy or even believe that they deserve their very much earned successes.

These impostors often view themselves as faking, 'bluffing' their way through their lives and undeserving of any success or related praise or rewards. In fact, because of the way they view themselves, success becomes a burden, having to 'maintain the imposture' as they see it, and living with the constant dread of exposure.

A trigger for neurotic imposture is often a strong tendency towards perfectionism. Perfectionists can fall into two categories. A 'benign' perfectionist is one whose perfectionism does not negatively impact on their life. They can be happy to take pleasure in their accomplishments and successes and, if they do encounter failure, do not fixate on it or let it become an obsession. 'Absolute' perfectionism is very different. An absolute perfectionist will set themselves goals that are almost impossible to achieve. They believe themselves not good enough, but often think that they can improve if they just keep working harder and harder. When, despite the extra work, they fall short of the impossible targets, they are then consumed with thoughts and behaviours that are self-defeating. This is similar to Clance's impostor cycle, and may result in the development of exhausting and mentally draining workaholic tendencies, in an attempt to attain the next set of almost impossibly high goals.

Outside observers can view in a negative way the tendency that neurotic impostors may have to downplay and deny their successes, seeing it as a kind of false humility, but this is not the case. The impostors do not believe they deserve the praise, and the act of minimising the truth of their abilities also act as another psychological protection measure, fulfilling the impulse to have a way out, an exit strategy in place. Success leads to the difficulty of trying to maintain that success and that standard and so failure begins to look an almost desirable outcome, at least to the subliminal mind. While nobody truly wishes to fail, the removal of expectations would provide a measure of relief. At times, the impostor's behaviour can actually bring about the failure that they fear and almost crave at the same time. The anxiety regarding their performance level becomes so intrusive that it can become almost self-destructive in relation to the particular task or even their entire career.

The symptoms of neurotic imposture as defined in the article are the fear of failure and conversely the fear of success, along with a tendency towards perfectionism, procrastination and workaholic tendencies.

* * * * *

## Impostor Syndrome

Dr. Valerie Young is recognised as one of the foremost experts on the subject of Impostor Syndrome, and is the author of 'The Secret Thoughts of Successful Women.' Despite the title, which on her website Dr. Young states was not her choice, she does recognise that impostor syndrome is not gender specific, despite the thoughts held by researchers earlier in the subject's study. What she does say in her description on the book's page on her site is that 'While the impostor syndrome is not unique to women, they are more likely to agonize over tiny mistakes and blame themselves for failure, see even constructive criticism as evidence of their shortcomings; and chalk up their accomplishments to luck rather than skill. When they do succeed, they think "Phew, I fooled 'em again." Perpetually waiting to be "unmasked" doesn't just drain a woman's energy and confidence. It can make her more risk-averse and less self-promoting than her male peers, which can hurt her future success.' More details of the book and Dr. Young's work can be read on her website.

Dr. Young defined five headings that each describe a personality type, patterns that seem to feed into impostor syndrome. Each personality type functions in a different way, but can all lead to the feelings of fraudulence and fakery with which sufferers struggle.

## The Perfectionist

The perfectionist sets themselves almost impossibly high goals and then, when they fail to achieve those goals, the result is a huge amount of self-doubt and the feeling that they are not good enough, that they do not measure up to their peers. This will not stop them setting the next targets just as much out of reach. The most important distinction that they consider is exactly how the assigned task is completed. Only absolute perfection is acceptable and any flaw is unacceptable. Any minor mistake, no matter how little impact it actually has on the final result, can cause feelings of failure and shame in the perfectionist.

The perfectionist can also often be the type of person who feels they have to be entirely in control, that the only way to have a task performed 'properly' is to do it themselves.

## The Expert

The expert feels a need to have a great amount of knowledge and ability to perform the required tasks, and it is the primary concern of their professional life. No matter how much they know and how many things they can do with competence, they always feel that it is not enough, will never be enough, and that they are pretenders compared to others who they assume must have a greater level of knowledge and ability. Any lack or gaps in their knowledge are marks of their lack of worth, and this denotes the sufferer as a failure in their own mind.

## The Soloist

This type of person feels that, if they cannot complete a task alone, without any help, they are not good enough. Any achievement is not a 'real' achievement unless they have managed to do it by themselves, no matter what or how much is involved. Needing any amount of advice or help at all is a sign of failure and lack of ability.

## The Natural Genius

This type of impostor syndrome sufferer feels that, unless they have an innate natural ability to perform a task to perfection without requiring much effort or education, they are a failure. If a task cannot be completed quickly and easily, then the 'natural genius' feels they are incompetent, and that any amount of hard effort is no alternative. Any need to struggle or put in hard work to gain mastery of a skill or a subject, or if the first effort is not successfully completed as absolutely perfect, is marked down in the sufferer's mind as a fail. This is further complicated by the fact that, in a similar way to the perfectionist type, the natural genius will set their goals to be almost unattainable, and consider themselves a failure when they cannot achieve them first time, effortlessly. Failure evokes shame, and doubting of their own abilities and worth.

## The Super-being

This type of personality feels a failure if they do not achieve total success in every part of their lives. Family, hobbies, work – all must be handled with efficiency and proficiency, and with next to no obvious effort. Their sense of self-worth is tied in to just how many tasks they can take on and complete perfectly at the same time. Inevitably they cannot manage to master everything but see those around them as managing to do so, making them feel a sense of phoniness compared to their 'genuine' high-achieving colleagues. Falling short in one of however many jobs they are trying to complete at once marks them as a failure in their own minds, no matter just how much they are juggling at once. While everybody else sees a success in someone managing so much, the sufferer can only dwell on the things that have not gone right thinking that this makes them a fraud, although this could not be further from the actual truth and they are in fact a perfectly competent individual.

The super-being often moves towards workaholic tendencies, working ever longer and harder in an attempt to 'measure up' although this only really functions as a mask, a way to create a smokescreen hiding their internally held insecurities from the world and, to a large extent, themselves. This move towards always working harder to make up for their perceived lack of talent can have serious implications for the sufferer's mental health and relationships with family and friends.

# THE CRITICAL INNER VOICE

One of the common signs of impostor syndrome – and one of the most difficult to combat – is something called the inner critic, or critical inner voice. This psychological term describes an internally located subpersonality that acts as a mental voice, making judgemental and demeaning comments about the person to whom it belongs. As the word critical implies, this voice does not promote positive thoughts, but rather concentrates on projecting negativity. The inner critic is not a benevolent entity but functions as rather more of an internal enemy, endangering the person's self-worth and their actions towards self-fulfilment. Often the opinions expressed by this inner voice invoke feelings of inadequacy, worthlessness and being wrong. They turn the focus inwards and focus on thoughts centred on self-criticism and self-denial. Because the voice is internal, there is no way to escape its effects without serious effort, and this can have effects on every part of the person from their state of mind, through their attitudes and their prejudices, and can go right through to having serious effects on their work performance. Constant exposure to these thoughts, altered moods, and emotions can result in a sense of shame and low self-esteem, both of which then encourage the critical inner voice to continue finding fault. The person struggling with their inner critic will repeatedly find they are caught up in thoughts of their own deficiencies and failings, leading to a greater extent of falling self-confidence and further doubting of their abilities, talents and worth. This can only have negative effects on mental health, and the debilitating effects can lead to the serious issues of anxiety and depression.

The effects of the critical inner voice can be seen in all areas of life, and can be particularly damaging to careers, as it can lead to the victim of the voice restricting their life to control the exposure to the negative thoughts. Refusing to take chances where things could potentially go wrong to lessen the opportunities the critical inner voice has to make its unpleasant presence known. This is understandable as, particularly due to its internal intrusive nature, it can affect almost every facet of the person's life. The way in which the voices criticises the self, damages self-worth and self-esteem and ravages the person's confidence in themselves can be hugely damaging to state of mind, relationships with others in professional and social settings, and professional performance. The thoughts can become self-fulfilling as, in an effort to quiet the thoughts, the sufferer changes the way in which they challenge themselves, and even lead to avoiding challenging themselves to keep developing. This can then make the problem worse again, as listening to those intrusive thoughts and following their advice can prompt further issues around self-esteem and self-worth, creating more of these thoughts and making the cycle worse.

# IMPOSTOR SYNDROME AND THE CANINE WORLD

The professional canine world is largely inhabited by incredibly passionate people and, as a result, it can be a very challenging world to be a part of. Divisions in thinking regarding methods and underlying thinking can be deep to say the least, and those divisions almost inevitably create a huge amount of discussion. These discussions can be amicable, but can also become deeply acrimonious and unpleasant between followers of rival thinking and methodologies. It only takes a mention of such words as 'dominance' or 'pack leader' for the atmosphere to heat up in a moment.

It is small wonder then that impostor syndrome does seem to be a common issue amongst canine professionals, particularly for those starting out on their journey into the professional canine world. Stepping out into that exposed arena to express an opinion can be intimidating at the best of times, and any self-doubt harboured in the mind will find ready ground to grow into a far bigger issue and unwillingness to stick your neck out and get involved. This really is truly understandable, but very soon puts a tight restriction on our ability to grow and develop as canine professionals who can effectively help and give advice to our clients, both canine and human.

The somewhat free-form nature of the paths that can be taken to become a canine professional are also a complicating factor. The industry is, as of writing, not under the control of any kind of official regulation and there are few requirements we need to satisfy to be able to call ourselves canine professionals. There are restrictions that have to be addressed to become a clinical behaviourist, for example, but to be able to work as a professional dog trainer or dog walker, there is no set path.

Excellent education is available from a number of sources, but the lack of defined requirements can lead to much disagreement about which education providers are best, which can feed into a process of second-guessing what you have learned and know. Some canine related education providers do not help the matter by attempting to disparage other companies. As with many categories of online and distance learning, the quality of course material, tutoring available, and customer service can vary wildly, and careful research is recommended when selecting which companies are worth studying with. The most expensive are not necessarily the best, as there are some great companies providing huge value for money with their educational offerings. It does pay to be initially dubious of canine course prices that seem too good to be true and it is always worth asking a few professional colleagues that you respect for their experiences with the companies they have chosen previously. Bear in mind also that we are all individuals. Preferences in learning styles will vary. This means that what suits one person may well not suit someone else well or at all.

Experience is also a huge part of being a canine professional and it is almost impossible to understate the value of practical hands on experience. This can be one of the challenges to confidence early in a canine professional career. Many wonderful and very experienced canine professionals are happy to mentor less experienced colleagues and help them to gain that experience in a constructive, safe, and ethical manner. If a perceived lack of practical experience is damaging confidence, try approaching some local well-regarded professionals about the possibility of shadowing some of their classes, or helping out. It may well seem intimidating to think of contacting respected professional people for such a purpose, but the gains from finding someone to learn from can be huge. Even the most experienced canine professional you can think of lacked experience at some point. The best of them went out despite any nerves they may have felt and found that route to practical experience, and the really good ones are often happy to help newer entrants in the same way.

If you have already gained the practical experience of doing your job as a canine professional but are still having huge issues with confidence, then it may be that impostor syndrome is to blame.

# FEAR OF FAILURE AND THE STRESS RESPONSE

One of the cruellest aspects of impostor syndrome is that for some, even the achievement of a successful result does not automatically mean a result of feeling happy. Because of the way in which impostor syndrome plays on the mind of the sufferer, success immediately provokes concerns about an ability to maintain that level of success with the attendant emotions of fear and self-doubt, and the sufferer will experience a level of discomfort concerning their achievements and the way that other people see them. All of these feed into a condition of living with stress. All of these feelings handicap the sufferer's ability to perceive accurately their abilities and achievements. When the sufferer comes up against a task that is based on achieving a certain result, the fear of failure will often trigger anxiety, sometimes to uncontrollable levels, which can have a severe negative effect on that person's psychological balance and well-being.

Although not an actual defined psychological condition, the effects of impostor syndrome on those living with it must not be under-estimated. Anticipating failure can cause a stress response, a series of biochemical and physical changes in the body. Fear, including fear of failure, involves some of the most ancient, primitive parts of the mammalian nervous system.

The nervous system has two sections: the central nervous system consisting of the brain and spinal cord, and the peripheral nervous system, the network of nerves running from the central nervous system throughout the body. These nerves feed information from the body in to the central nervous system and relay any required instructions back out to the relevant body parts.

The peripheral nervous system splits into three parts:

• the somatic nervous system, which deals with matters under the conscious control, such as muscle movements.
• the enteric nervous system, which is not often discussed and is situated in the digestive system. It consists of a mesh of nerve fibres throughout the gastrointestinal system.
• the autonomic nervous system, which deals

with things not under the body's conscious control, including digestion, respiration, heart rate, and the stress response.

The autonomic nervous system splits again into a further two divisions.

The parasympathetic nervous system deals with that is colloquially known as the 'rest and digest' functions, what happens in the body when everything is fine and normal. This normal condition is known as homeostasis, and the parasympathetic division is responsible for returning the body to homeostasis after a stressful situation, and then maintaining that condition.

The other side of the division, the 'fight or flight' side, more properly known as the sympathetic nervous system, is what moves into action when a situation is considered stressful, such as worrying about completing an achievement related task.

In a stressful situation, the amygdala – an almond-shaped structure in the brain's temporal lobe involved in the processing of emotions – sets the hypothalamus into action. The hypothalamus sits near the base of the brain and, although small, it is an important part of many functions in the body including:

• appetite control
• emotional response regulation

- managing sexual behaviour
- regulating body temperature
- hormone release

The hypothalamus sends signals within the brain to the pituitary gland, which is also known as the body's master gland. This is because it produces hormones that control other glands in the body, such as the thyroid, adrenal, and reproductive glands. The pituitary gland produces a hormone called ACTH (adrenocorticotropic hormone). This hormone, together with a signal from the hypothalamus, stimulates the adrenal glands located on the kidneys. The adrenal medulla – the inner part of the gland – in response produces adrenaline. Chemical messengers on the blood also prompt the adrenal cortex on the outside of the adrenal gland to produce cortisol.

This process as a response to fear is designed to put the body into a state ready to survive the immediate situation. A number of changes prepare the system to be able to run or fight the way out of a situation as required:

- the liver provides glucose into the bloodstream for extra energy if required.
- increased blood pressure
- increased heart rate
- stronger and more forceful heart contractions
- pupils dilate
- reduced blood flow through constricted blood vessels to the urinary and gastrointestinal

systems, slowing urine production and digestive activity
• energy usually directed to immune system function is redirected to prepare for the fight or flight response
• dilated bronchioles in the lungs increase breathing capacity and oxygen uptake
• respiration rate increases

Adrenaline produced in the body during a stress response can clear the body fast, within a matter of minutes after the situation has been resolved. Cortisol takes longer, from a few hours to a couple of days or more according to some studies. Once the stress hormones have dissipated, the parasympathetic system steps in to restore the body to the 'rest and digest' state and baseline normal status, also known as homeostasis.

In the short term, fear is a natural and healthy response to something threatening in the environment. When the body has a chance to recover from the effects of the hormones, no kind of lasting harm is done. Living with long-term stress means that this is not able to happen.

As previously mentioned, cortisol can take some time to leave the body. If, due to chronic stress, cortisol levels are not able to return to baseline levels, a number of issues can arise in and for the stressed individual. From a biological perspective, the fear response is meant to be a short-term state, a matter of survival that of short duration. It is not designed to be running on high alert for long periods, known as chronic stress, such as worrying about not measuring up at work, as in impostor syndrome.

The stress response diverts the body's resources away from the systems regarded as not essential during an immediate survival situation. These include the digestive, reproductive, urinary, and immune systems. While all of the described suppressions make sense in the short term, the difficulties posed by having these systems not functioning properly for an extended period are detrimental to health. The issues around lacking a properly working immune system are easy to see.

With the way the digestive and urinary systems are not functioning as they should, a body under constant stress often feels sick and tired. To combat tiredness, the body naturally wants to sleep more but elevated stress levels mean sleep becomes elusive and so making the stressed person more tired. This creates a vicious cycle which can lead to a number of potentially serious health conditions such as problems with the kidneys, and cardiovascular disease, including heart disease, high blood pressure, and abnormal heart rhythms. All of these can make the person feel even more ill and vulnerable, adding to the stress and making the situation yet again worse.

The links between impostor syndrome and psychological distress as a consequence, including anxiety and depression, have been identified for some time. The experience of living with impostor syndrome, and the effects of existing with an ongoing level of long-term stress can come together in a set of subclinical psychological symptoms that, if they are not addressed, can lead to a clinical level case of anxiety and/or depression.

## SIGNS OF IMPOSTOR SYNDROME

A number of signals are defined that can point to a case of impostor syndrome. The overriding feeling found is inadequacy, no matter how successful you might be in your life and career, and a sense of fraudulence, that you are tricking the people around you into believing you are competent. For some sufferers, continued success only doubles down on these feelings, adding in a sense of dread to daily life, as they fear discovery, being 'outed' as a fake, or simply lucky to have achieved what they have. A number of common thoughts might point towards realising that you suffer from impostor syndrome. These thoughts can, to the sufferer, seem perfectly rational although the underlying assertions are in fact completely irrational and not based in truth.

## If I can do it, it must be easy

If the impostor syndrome sufferer finds a task

easy compared to other people, they tend to think that anyone can do it. If it is easy for them, it must be easy for everyone. Those with impostor syndrome often devalue their own unique combinations of abilities, talents, and gifts. If comments are made by others about how well something has been done, these will be downplayed, deflected and dismissed as not being accurate.

## I'm a total fake

Sufferers feel that they do not deserve any of the praise or accolades that they receive. Their view is that they have managed to fool the people around them into thinking they are talented and competent. They live convinced that somebody is going to realise, is going to find them out and everyone will know they are a fraud.

## It's all down to luck

Successes are written off as being due to luck or being in the right place at the right time. They do not believe that any success they have could be down to their skills, talents or abilities.

## It wasn't just me, I had help.

Sufferers can phrase things in their own minds that any help or support received from colleagues or friends negates their own input into the task and so any positive feedback is written off as being because of the others involved.

## I must not fail

If a task results in failure, the sufferer thinks that will mean everyone realising they were no good all along and they are incompetent, rather than accepting that everyone makes mistakes and things go wrong sometimes. They cannot see failure as something to learn from for future tasks, but fear it as the worst thing that could happen. This also feeds into the vicious cycle of impostor syndrome as, if they achieve success in the current task, the pressure is increased further for subsequent tasks as there is a deep and urgent need to keep the success going to avoid being 'found out' by their peers. This fear of discovery can push people to work right up to the limit of their capacity, attempting to prevent their employers or colleagues exposing what they see as their fraudulence and lack of competence. Despite the extra effort they go to trying to prevent this, they will still not see their efforts as being enough, adding in to the vicious cycle that impostor syndrome can create and creating further issues around lowered self-confidence, self-esteem and fostering self-doubt.

# If it's not difficult to achieve, it can't really be worthwhile

Those with impostor syndrome struggle to recognise their own talents, or to believe that what they might find easy others can find difficult. They can sometimes invent factors to complicate the task, making it more 'worthwhile' in a form of self-handicapping and making the current task more difficult. This becomes self-fulfilling as the sufferer piles on ever more complicating factors to make the task more 'worthwhile' and, in the end, that task might become unachievable. In adding the extra issues required to complete the current task, in some ways the person is setting up a kind of cushion, a safety net in that they have these extra factors they can point to as a reason they failed and could not complete the job. Failing is still a major issue for this person, but the protection of the complicating factors can take some of the sting out of failing, as they can point to that as making it not entirely their fault failure occurred. The longer this continues the more exhausting it becomes and the more important it is that the cycle is broken.

# No amount of achievement is ever enough

Impostor syndrome sufferers can set themselves standards that are virtually impossible to maintain consistently. They compare themselves to others and, no matter how much they have actually achieved, they do not see themselves as equally successful and worthy of praise. They place themselves in a position where they become almost their own competition, as they are fighting against themselves more to feel accomplished and competent in their careers than they are against any external competition. This can be particularly difficult in people who place an incredibly high value on external validation. No matter how many positive reviews they receive, they are looking hungrily for that next confidence boost of positive feedback. If coupled with almost entirely unattainable standards, this is a combination that is bound to lead to disappointment and a drop in self-esteem and perception of self-worth.

## Focusing on the negatives

Instead of recognising and acknowledging their positive impact on the world and those around them, their clients and peers, those with impostor syndrome can dwell for a long time on any kind of mistake or failure. Rather than seeing all of the things they have managed to achieve and to do well, the slightest thing that could have gone wrong takes all of their focus and becomes magnified out of all proportion. This negative focus can be so consistent that it becomes a habit. The nagging, constant sense of fear and anxiety comes to feel like out natural state.

## Play it safe, to a huge degree

In an attempt to avoid failure, and because they believe they just aren't good enough to achieve more, sufferers can stop challenging themselves and stretching their boundaries. It is an attempt at a form of self-protection, but becomes a kind of self-sabotage as the avoidance of stretching those boundaries can be damaging to their career growth.

## All I can think about is the fear

If we are focusing too hard on the fear and anxiety that impostor syndrome so often causes, our thoughts are not on the job that we need to concentrate on. This shift of thinking to a non-constructive slant can take us straight out of the moment, and remove our focus and ability to concentrate on the things we really need to be thinking about to get the project underway or the job finished. When the experience of being overwhelmed by the emotions blocks our ability to be able to function and concentrate on the practical as necessary, this can easily lead to failure, and an increase to the fear and anxiety when approaching the next new project or task.

A particular difficulty with impostor syndrome that complicates the matter is that it can be very difficult to recognise in yourself. Many people that struggle with impostor syndrome can easily identify others as exhibiting it. When it comes to themselves, they will still believe that they are genuinely impostors, and really are less competent than they have persuaded others to perceive them as being.

# WHAT CAUSES IMPOSTOR SYNDROME?

The short answer is that there is no single, simple answer.

The causal mechanisms of impostor syndrome have not been fully defined. We do not have something that we can definitively say is the cause of impostor syndrome. A number of the experts who have studied the phenomenon think it is linked with certain personality traits, including anxiety and neuroticism. Others believe it can come from behavioural causes or traced back to events in the family history. A number of studies have associated it as correlating in a proportion of cases with growing up having over-protective parents. Higher levels of perceived parental control coupled with low self-esteem levels corresponded frequently with impostor fears, seeming to be a possible notable predictor of impostor syndrome. There are also researchers that have studied impostor syndrome who have theorised a connection with families who value achievement to a very high degree, or where the parents/caregivers veered between high levels of praise and criticism, giving no solid framework in which they can learn to assess reliably their abilities and achievements. Common theories are that impostor syndrome can develop from childhood memories centred around this inconsistency of praise and criticism from authority figures, being eclipsed by siblings or led in some other way to feel that you are not good enough and don't measure up.

External factors unconcerned with personality traits are also thought to play a role. The environments in which we put ourselves have a huge effect on us, and spending time in negative environments can have a huge ongoing effect in our lives and minds. Another potential major factor is institutionalised discrimination. Early in the history of research into impostor syndrome, it was originally thought to only affect women. While it is now known this is not the case, it does seem that women are more prone, although anyone in a significant minority for some reason in their professional world can suffer with impostor syndrome.

So now we know how to recognise impostor syndrome, how do we go about stopping it interfering with our lives as canine professionals? The most important factor in helping to stop feeling like an impostor is to reframe your thoughts so that you are no longer thinking like an impostor. Impostor syndrome is not an inevitable part of professional life, it can be avoided and its effects lessened.

# CONQUERING THE INNER CRITIC

The first step in quieting that inner critic, the insistent internal voice telling you that you are not good enough, is to identify exactly what it is telling you. To be able to tackle the negative thoughts this inner critic is filling our heads with to hold us back, the first thing to do is to identify them. To do this, think about the areas of life, e.g. professional skills and knowledge, that the inner critic is particularly prone to attacking, and then identify the specific criticisms. It can be useful to write them down for the purposes of identification and realising which aspects of confidence need working on.

To take some of the sting out of the negative thoughts that can make dealing with them and progressing, try phrasing them in the second person. Instead of 'I don't have the knowledge to help people with their dogs' try thinking something like 'You don't have the knowledge' instead. The thought is no less false, but removing the direct connection can help make it feel less personal and start to allow the sufferer to get the thoughts under control.

Recognising the origin of the critical thoughts is very useful to helping overcome them. There is thought to be some correlation between growing up in an atmosphere framed in highly critical feedback, or in a family with a very successful sibling, in terms of praise from caregivers if not in fact. Once the obvious unfairness is balanced out by effort at reasoned thought when removed from the injurious environment, the lack of truth in the criticisms is easier to see.

Once the thoughts projected by the critical inner voice have been identified and categorised in the above ways, examine how they cause your behaviour to change. Once you understand how these intrusive thoughts manipulate how you do things, you can begin to see how to change those behaviour patterns and eliminate the negative effects of the inner critic's assertions.

Start to disrupt the hold that the inner critic holds on you by not engaging in the kind of self-destructive behaviours that the critical inner voice encourages. The more a sufferer can increase their use of positive behaviours that go against the negative recommendations of the voice, the weaker its grip will become. A common kind of self-sabotage that the inner critic persuades a sufferer to partake in is sitting back in discussions and not taking part, even though their level of knowledge, experience and abilities mean they are perfectly qualified to contribute. The more that person can bring themselves to actively take part in discussions involving their area of knowledge, the more they can begin to see that what the inner critic is telling them is wrong.

It sounds very simple, this process of realising that the false inner critic exists, identifying the false thoughts they project and turning thinking around to a more positive mindset. The theory is indeed simple, but the act of following it through can be much harder than it seems. Change is often something that people can find hard, and tackling things that require change can sometimes lead to anxiety. This is particularly true for situations in which the sufferers already doubt themselves to any kind of extent, because the inner critic has its claws into them from the beginning. The situation can feel worse before it starts to feel better. To manage to defeat the inner critic, perseverance is the key. If the sufferer wants to stop the negative thoughts holding them back, they need to keep going, framing their world using positive thoughts and making sure they are embracing that continuing positivity. The more they follow the process and do embrace that positive thinking, the weaker the influence of the inner critic becomes, freeing that person from the restrictions their mind put on them and enabling them to go on and achieve goals that the inner critic would never have let them imagine possible, living life without those negative limitations.

This mindset of perseverance that can conquer the inner critic is also key for combatting any form of impostor syndrome. Once the sufferer begins to realise that success is possible, that they can achieve what they set out to do, and can start to string a series of positive, successful experiences together, the expectations of results can change. From automatic assumption that failure will happen, the beginnings of anticipating success can creep in. It is unlikely to be a quick process, as impostor syndrome by its nature is very persistent, and involves a kind of cycle that is very difficult from which to break free. Perseverance really is key.

# COMBATTING IMPOSTOR SYNDROME IN PERSONALITY TYPES

In an earlier section of this book, we had a look at the definitions of some categories of personality types seen in impostor syndrome types written about by Dr. Valerie Young. If you can recognise one of these personality types as applying to you, there are some specific tools and ideas to combat each different type.

## The Perfectionist

The perfectionist needs to learn to live with the fact that humans make mistakes sometimes, and that making a mistake does not automatically make them failures. Expecting your work to be utterly flawless every single time is unrealistic. Once you can begin to accept that, life starts to become a little less stressful. Another aspect of beating the perfectionist tendency is to push yourself to try new things, before waiting to feel ready. This goes against the perfectionist tendency to feel they need to know everything about the subject or task before starting to work on it. This can be damaging to career progression as it can lead to putting off starting new projects and trying new things. The reality is that waiting for the 'perfect time' could mean never starting something new, as the perfect time will never come.

## The Super-being

The idea that success comes from hard work can lead to workaholic tendencies, and a kind of addiction to work and the validation that brings. A way to tackle this is to remove your concept of what success actually is away from the concept of external validation. Train yourself to assess how you feel about your work and achievements. Begin to empower yourself by focusing on the thought that nobody has the complete power over you to make you feel good or bad about yourself, and that constructive criticism is not a bad thing, but is a tool to help you learn and grow. That sense of self can help to balance the desire for external validation. Learning to concentrate on internal validation will aid your self-confidence and allow you to begin gauging how much work is actually required to achieve success. It can also help you to work out if your targets are being set too high for anyone to be able to reach them consistently.

# The Natural Genius

Nobody knows everything, and everybody has to learn something for the first time at some point. Some things may come to you easily, but others are likely to need a little more time to get to grips with. This does not mean that you are bad at them, or that you are never going to be any good at them. We are all works in progress. To be really good at something, including working with and understanding dogs, requires an ongoing learning process. As science progresses and never ends, so the learning and skill gathering processes never end either. Even the most accomplished and confident people you see in the dog world are likely to be continuing to expand their knowledge and skill sets. This is the function of CPD and the mark of a good professional – one that realises they don't and can't know everything, and keeps themselves up to date with scientific and ethical thinking surrounding dogs.

# The Soloist

To be successful and good at your job, it really is not necessary to do everything on your own. If you prefer to be independent, that is absolutely fine, but do not let it overtake your life to the point that you become isolated and refuse to accept help if you need it in a misguided attempt to 'prove your worth.' The truth is that, if you refuse ever to think about asking for help, you are most likely only going to slow down your own progression and growth as a professional.

## The Expert

Again, nobody knows everything. Increasing your knowledge and skillset is a valuable investment in your professional future, especially as new methods and approaches to dog training and handling come to your attention, and any developing business or licensing requirements come into place. Staying current professionally is important, but it is also important not to take it too far, so that you delay putting new ideas and projects into action because of the need you feel to know everything before starting. It is a form of procrastination. Learning is good, but it can be more constructive to practice learning on a just-in-time basis, adding extra skills as you need them rather than hoarding skills far in advance to the detriment of your career by not practising the skills you have previous gathered. It is also important to realise that asking for help is not shameful. In fact mentoring, whether as the one mentored or the one providing the mentoring, can give a massive boost to confidence.

## COMBATTING IMPOSTOR SYNDROME OUTSIDE OF PERSONALITY TYPES

If you do not recognise yourself in one of those categories, how do you go about combatting impostor syndrome? A number of tips and techniques are available that can help.

## Recognise the problem

The first step in dealing with a problem is recognising that you have a problem, and this is every bit as true for impostor syndrome as it is for any other issue. The good news is that if you are reading this book then the chances are you have started to cover this step already. Recognising those intrusive thoughts as the fake assertions of impostor syndrome is the first part of the process of removing their influence and power over you.

## Everyone goes through it at some time

Remember that everyone feels unsure and out of their depth at some points. It is human nature to feel concerned about trying something new for the first time, and the most confident and competent seeming people that you know have likely struggled with their confidence at some time. The important thing is to realise that those thoughts do not automatically have power over you. They do not have to control your life.

## Nobody's perfect

Remove the pressure to be perfect. Make sure that the goals you set for yourself are sufficiently challenging to keep your experience levels, knowledge, and career expanding, but are also realistic and achievable. Accept that mistakes are an inevitable part of being human, and we all make them from time to time. There is no shame in making mistakes, and they often provide some of our best learning opportunities. Strive to be competent and capable rather than perfect, and use any mistakes you do make as learning experiences that will help you to avoid that mistake and perform better on future occasions.

## Healthy work/life balance

It is really important to maintain a healthy work/life balance. Workaholic tendencies are not healthy, and it is important that worries and anxieties about work are not permitted to invade every area of life. Taking time to switch off from work and relax, letting your body and brain recover from any stresses connected with work is vital for physical and mental well-being. This can be difficult if you are working for yourself, running your own business, or working as a manager in charge of other people. It is very important to create boundaries to separate work and home life, as otherwise it can be very easy for work to take over life, starting in small imperceptible steps that build until work is occupying a large portion of your home and/or family time. Make sure that you make time for yourself, your family and friends in your life. The old saying of 'All work and no play makes Jack a dull boy' could more accurately be said as 'All work and no play damages Jack's health and well-being, mentally and physically,' which is both far clumsier to say, and a far more worrying prospect. If switching off is difficult, finding a hobby that is not connected with work and that occupies the brain in a way unconnected with your career can be useful to aid in that.

## Acknowledge the experience

Acknowledge the thoughts that you are experiencing. Awareness is a good thing and worrying about your performance shows that you care about your career. Consider creating an appraisal of yourself as a person and as a professional, writing down your areas of strength and weaknesses. When it comes to assessing yourself and beginning to work out just where the negative feelings associated with impostor syndrome come from, you are the best-placed person to know the source. Once you have objectively identified your strengths and weaknesses, you can already begin to feel more confident because you can see what you are good at, and what can be addressed and improved. The understanding of your abilities and weaknesses immediately removes them as such a factor to worry about because you know the qualifications and experience you have to do the job in front of you.

Once you have a list of the things you feel you need to work on and areas that you need to think about and come to terms with, you can start to deal with them. This may mean seeing that they are part of the pattern of creating fake thoughts, whether they are affecting areas in which you actually have experience or training, or realising they are things that you need to come to terms with and refuse to let have any further influence over you. Seeing the facts written objectively is a good tool to act as a reality check, and may well help you to see that you are far more qualified to do your job, and more experienced than many other people would be.

## The power of perspective

Context and perspective are important. Worrying about performance or being nervous about a new task or starting a new strand to your business is not automatically a problem. Feeling out of your depth for a while at the start of a new project is absolutely normal and fine. If the feelings are not persistent and pervasive, and there is a contextually valid reason for that feeling of concern, then that worry is not a problem. It is vital to be sure that we do not add worrying about being worried to the list of things that can trigger impostor syndrome. If you find yourself feeling anxious, take a moment to breathe and to check the context. If that valid reason is there, keep moving on. If that context is lacking, start working on switching your thinking to the positive.

## Identify cognitive coping mechanisms

Be aware of any coping strategies you might use in an attempt to protect yourself from failure. If you avoid starting new projects, or you have a tendency towards holding back from voicing opinions in group discussions or giving clients your opinions on matters that can help their dogs, these things need tackling. Although it is very difficult in the beginning, introduce the new project. Give the client the useful information. Take part in the discussion. If you have an opinion or an idea that could work, speak up. You have as much right to be heard in the area of your expertise as any other canine professional.

# Record positives

Keeping a journal and writing down the positive things that happen in a day can be a powerful thing to look back on when you are having a time where you are struggling. Keeping a record of positive feedback can also provide a real boost to remove the power of these thoughts. Whether you keep a record digitally or as a hard copy, when you are having a tough time, take a minute to read through some of the positive reviews you have received from others to give yourself an injection of confidence and a feel good factor.

# Be kind to yourself

Everyone makes mistakes from time to time. The key lies in learning to forgive yourself for your mistakes, and becoming able to frame them as an opportunity for a learning experience. Reframe the situations that have not gone to plan into learning opportunities and use the experiences you gain from things going a little wrong for whatever reason to improve your techniques and approaches for the future.

# Avoid comparison

If you have a tendency to compare yourself to others around you, and frequently find yourself feeling miserable as you perceive them as being 'better' than you in some or a number of ways, this is something that needs to stop. Focus on switching from needing external validation so strongly and find ways to use internal validation as a measure of how happy you are with your performance. By sticking to focusing on yourself, concentration moves to the things that you can have an effect on, the things that you can control. You cannot influence how well others do their job in comparison to you, so comparing has little effectiveness and less positive influence on your mindset or performance. Concentrate on being happy with your own performance, and how you do your job, and on the things you can control.

## Redefine your perceptions of failure

Many suffering with impostor syndrome have very strong tendencies towards perfectionism. Anything less than an immaculate completion of a task or project is viewed as a failure. Sufferers need to learn to accept that mistakes happen. Nobody knows everything. Nobody can automatically do everything to a perfect standard. Not knowing something or not knowing how to do something is not a failure. Making a mistake and getting something wrong does not mean that your professional life is a lie and that you are a fraud, a fake or not worthy of calling yourself a professional. When things go wrong, as they inevitably do for everyone at times, do not let yourself dwell on it or let it fester inside, poisoning your self-confidence, self-esteem and self-worth. If you make a mistake, take the lessons that you need from it so that you can feel confidence that particular error or mistake will not happen again. If you get a little stuck because of something you do not know, seek out that knowledge so that you are prepared next time. Do not let anything make you be afraid to try new things, as that can stunt your career growth and progress.

## Reward yourself

Positive reinforcement is scientifically proven to be the best motivation possible in training dogs, and it works for people too! When you have had a success in a task, for example your new training class has proved to be a hit, or you get some great positive feedback from a client, allow yourself to accept and absorb that positive feeling and treat yourself to something you find rewarding, because you have earned it.

## Visualise success

Use visualisation to aid in keeping you feeling calm and able to focus constructively on the task at hand. Imagining yourself successfully completing a task can have a strong influence on your mindset, pushing you towards a more positive frame of mind. Positivity and positive thinking is one of the greatest tools in the battle against impostor syndrome. Kind, effective, and ethical dog people are used to framing their thinking around dogs in a positive way. Extending that way of thinking to be kind to ourselves, and think of ourselves in that positive way, removes some of the stress and pressure we put on ourselves.

## Focus on the positives

As well as visualisations, work on reframing thoughts into positives instead of negatives. Instead of thinking 'I can't do this, I'm not good enough or clever enough,' try to think positively along the lines of 'I can do this, I am able. I have the right skills and talents to do this.' If that is a step too far in the early stages of combatting your impostor syndrome then, rather than focusing on the negative, try thinking 'I might feel useless at the moment, but that does not mean that the thoughts are right, or that I am useless.' Reframing thoughts in a way that removes any self-doubt contained in them immediately starts to take out the chances of feeling like an impostor. Positive thinking holds a massive amount of power over our mental states. When you manage to complete a task successfully, allow yourself to absorb the feeling of achievement and accomplishment and build on it towards the positive thinking.

## Accept and acknowledge your self-worth

If accepting praise and compliments does not come easily to you, practice. Go to the record of positive feedback mentioned earlier and read some of the good reviews or appraisals you have received in the past. Practice internalising that success, letting yourself absorb it and realising that it is the truth of you and your work. When new feedback or praise comes, do not let yourself deflect it by claiming external factors are the reason for your success. If someone is telling you how well you have done, accept the praise and believe that you deserve it. It may be how much difference you have made to their life by improving their relationship with their dog, for instance, or helping the human client to understand how to work on changing a behaviour. Finding the perfect walks for a client's anxious dog so that they are happy, chilled, and relaxed at home. That person is telling you what a great job you have done because they know you are the one responsible for the good things that have happened. Let yourself accept that the person who came to you needing help and advice is well placed to know who is the one that succeeded in giving them the help, advice, knowledge, or services that they really needed.

## Expand your boundaries

One of the most restrictive things about impostor syndrome is the way in which it can prevent sufferers from trying new things and adding new strands to their skillsets, and new services to their businesses. Although this is incredibly hard to contemplate when you are at the beginning of trying to take control of your impostor syndrome, pushing yourself out of your comfort zone once rational thought says that you are ready will result in increased confidence. When you begin to prove the negative thoughts wrong and demonstrate that you can do the new thing it can give you confidence to carry on doing more new things.

## Fight the fear

Following on from the above point, try taking the advice of Susan Jeffers, the author of 'Feel the Fear and Do It Anyway.' Lean into the fear and do not let it control your life. Lean into that fear and lack of confidence and push through it. Working through a problem or task despite the trepidation surrounding it can give your self-esteem a massive boost. The more you try and manage to do successfully, the more you can learn to believe in your abilities and skills to be able to deal with whatever your human or canine clients send in your direction.

## Don't suffer in silence

In a 1978 paper, Clance and Imes described a therapeutic approach they used in their clinical setting and with the women in their initial study on impostor phenomenon. They proposed that it could be effective as a tool to help those suffering with the problem. Included in their technique is the use of group therapy, gathering sufferers together to discuss and relate their experiences together. A number of researchers stated that the group sessions helped the participants, and that the ability for an individual to realise that they are not the only one experiencing impostor syndrome can help negate the effects on them.

An alternative to group therapy that can be effective and is easier to access is to seek support from others. This can include friends, family and colleagues in the work or business world. Sharing the experience of these negative thoughts can help as the sufferer discovers others that feel the same way, or can calm the negative thoughts around perceptions of the sufferer's abilities by their peers. Find a place where you feel safe to talk, whether in person or online, and talk about how you feel and your struggles with the negative intrusive thoughts. There is a very strong chance that when you do this you will find others experiencing exactly the same issues. You can then all come together to provide help and support for each other, all battling the issues together. An open dialogue with others is much healthier and more constructive than suffering alone. If you talk to somebody that you respect and trust to be honest about your abilities and skill level, they can show you that your fears of being incompetent are unfounded, or help you to identify the areas that you can work on, and come up with a plan on how to do so.

# Find support

While the canine professional world can be a difficult place to inhabit due to its sometimes fractious and divisive nature, there are some wonderful kind and supportive people in that world as well. If you can find someone who you respect to act as a mentor it can hugely help your confidence, and aid in giving you a sense of perspective of just how skilled and valuable you are as a canine professional. Finding a mentor that you respect and trust means you have a professional who you can ask for help to work out where you might benefit from developing aspects of your education and skills, and can also help you to make an accurate assessment of yourself. If your mentor states that, no matter how much you might see yourself as inadequate and less than competent, they see a qualified, experienced and capable professional, that gives an independent indication that your opinions of your professional value and worth is not based in truth. Finding support in a group of peers can also be incredibly helpful and, when you have begun to get your impostor syndrome contained, you can pay it forward by supporting others in that group or becoming a mentor to others yourself. Helping others in the same situation as you can also help you see how the impostor thinking does not represent the real professional you.

## Positivity breeds positivity

There is nothing wrong with being selective of the people with whom you choose to spend your time, especially when dealing with an issue like impostor syndrome. Choosing to be around people who lift you up as much as you can will aid in making your entire mindset more positive. The more positive environment has beneficial effects on your mental state and well-being, which plays a massive part in being able to accept yourself as you are.

## Assess how you use social media

Interacting with online communities can be a hugely positive thing, and in many cases is an almost vital part of marketing yourself as a professional in modern times. There can be a real temptation to use the distance that social media places between us by all being behind a separate device screen to project an image of yourself as different to your reality. Whether this is because that image does not match who you really are, or it plays into projecting a standard that would be impossible for you to achieve, trying to keep that false image going can only make things worse. Use social media carefully and stick firmly to the objective truth of your situation, knowledge and experience.

# Fake it till you make it

Talking about faking it may seem like a strange thing to write in a text that is dealing with the mental condition of permanently feeling like a bit of a fake. In this case faking it refers to confidence. What we practice becomes truth. When you push yourself to take that step of taking part in a discussion on your area of knowledge and experience, or start that new project that you have planned carefully, and do so with an air of confidence, the results will be positive. This gives a great platform to carry on growing in confidence, as you begin to realise that you do know these things and can do that task, that confidence will only increase and percolate through all areas of your life.

# Take things one step at a time

When working on areas that you have objectively calculated do need further study or practice, do not pressure yourself to perform them perfectly. Work out what it takes to complete tasks reasonably well without demanding too much in the early stages, and look to improve performance gradually if necessary. Make sure to reward yourself for actually taking action, as this is a huge step towards reducing the impact impostor syndrome can have on your life.

# See the constructive in constructive criticism

Learn to accept constructive criticism. It does not mean that you are not good at what you do. Constructive criticism gives us a framework that we can use to improve our professional skills and identify areas of skillset or knowledge that would benefit from being expanded or practiced further. Try not to take this constructive criticism personally, as it is not directed at you as a person, but shows where you as a professional entity can improve.

## Find a well-rounded balance

Impostor syndrome makes it very difficult for sufferers to accept their successes and the praise, accolades, and compliments that come with success. They downplay and deflect, attributing their success to external factors rather than their own abilities, skills, and talents, including help from others, luck, or fortunate timing, among others. Any mistakes or errors, on the other hand, are soon internalised and they blame themselves, frequently for an extended period of time. Indeed, some people suffering with impostor syndrome can hang on to what others would dismiss as a minor error for far longer than could be considered healthy, in some cases for years.

Any mistakes that are made do need to be absorbed and acknowledged, but not lingered over to the exclusion of seeing the good that you manage to achieve. The aim should be to acquire a well-rounded attitude to mistakes and success. Do not dwell on the mistakes but see what went wrong and what can be done better next time. Once this has happened, move on.

Equally, when you have a success, it is vital to acknowledge your abilities and skills that allowed the success to happen. Realise it, accept it, own it. Learn to accept the praise and positive feedback that comes with success. Do not write successes off to luck. Remember what Arnold Palmer, regarded as one of the greatest and most charismatic golfers of all time, said about luck. 'It's a funny thing, the more I practice, the luckier I get.' What you regard as luck is quite likely the results of the effort you have put into increasing your learning and expanding your skillset and experience level. The more you let yourself absorb the successes, and acknowledge that it is not luck but your effort, experience, and education that have made the success happen, the more comfortable you will become with your talents, skills, and knowledge level, and the less trepidation will be involved in your professional life.

## Keep on keeping on

Getting past impostor syndrome is not quick and it is not easy. It take time and work. That effort and the hours spent putting the plans to deal with the negative thoughts into action will be worth it in the end. The best way to beat impostor syndrome is to keep on working towards your goals no matter what the impostor syndrome is trying to tell you. The more you can keep going and successfully managing despite what the thoughts are saying in your head, the more evidence you are building to disprove their assertions. There are some people for whom more successes can pile further pressure on to maintain a level of performance, but by working with the advice contained in this book to mitigate the power of negative thoughts, they can be got under better control. Success can then breed confidence, and when you can start to build up your confidence, then you can achieve even more, meaning that you can begin to build the career you really want, unhampered by those negative thoughts.

# COGNITIVE RESTRUCTURING

Another tool that can be very powerful in tackling impostor syndrome is the use of cognitive restructuring and positive affirmations. This can help with learning to take the intrusive negative thoughts that impostor syndrome feeds in so insidiously and replace them with positive based statements. This allows for those negative thoughts to be neutralised with the positive affirmations. In the process of working though combatting impostor syndrome utilising this approach, cognitive restructuring follows on from recognising and acknowledging the feelings of fraudulence, which is the first step in every method.

The American Psychological Association's Dictionary of Psychology defines automatic thoughts as:

"1. Thoughts that are instantaneous, habitual, and nonconscious. Automatic thoughts affect a person's mood and actions. Helping individuals to become aware of the presence and impact of negative automatic thoughts, and then to test their validity, is a central task of cognitive therapy.

2. Thoughts that have been so well learned and habitually repeated that they occur without cognitive effort. Also called routinized thoughts."

To employ cognitive restructuring and deal with the habitual input of these distorted negative automatic thoughts that becomes the default setting for those with impostor syndrome, there are a number of steps to follow:

• Take a few moments to calm and try to find a sense of mental balance.

• Define what is going on.

• Identify the moods felt as the situation occurs. Moods are not thoughts. This is an important distinction, as moods link to the fundamental basic emotions. A simple way to differentiate moods from thoughts is that a mood only needs a single word to describe it (sad, nervous, angry, worried for example) while to identify thoughts requires a much more complex description.

• Note down the reactions you experienced when the mood occurred. These natural reactions are also known as automatic thoughts.

• Look for evidence that objectively supports those automatic thoughts and then evidence that objectively disproves the thoughts. The idea behind this is to gain an objective view of the situation, and see what happened that kicked off the automatic thoughts and prompted the negative feelings that impostor syndrome brings. The second lot of objective evidence, the one that disproves those thoughts, is where rational thought begins to enter the process, as opposed to behaviours based on pure reactions.

• Once you have examined both sides and have the supporting and contradictory evidence for those thoughts, the situation can be analysed in a fair and balanced way. This removes the reactive emotional response and allows more of an objective view of the whole situation. If things still feel unclear to you, it may be a good idea to ask a person you trust and respect to talk it through with you, or find a different way to look at things and test the question until you have a balanced view noted down to work with.

• Now the immediate stress of the situation has dissipated and there has been time to think about it calmly, take a moment to assess your current mood. With that distance from the emotional kneejerk of the stressful situation, mood should usually have much improved. As long as this is the case it is now time to think about the situation, and what you can do to change things in the future.

Once this process is complete it is time to begin creating some positive thoughts and statements to counter the negative automatic thoughts the next time that kind of situation arises again.

## Positive affirmations

Positive affirmations are short statements, maybe one or two sentences, designed to be repeated frequently to yourself as a counter to any negative automatic thoughts and feelings that may habitually arise. Created and repeated to encourage and inspire the person saying or thinking them, they have the function of deflecting chances to self-sabotage until they have worked to the extent that there are no longer such strong self-sabotaging thoughts interfering with the ability to tackle tasks confidently. With continued repetition, the mental position switches to believing these statements and replacing the negative automatic thoughts with positive ones. With repeated use of positive affirmations, the patterns of our thoughts can alter to provide a more positive outlook and framework. As the positivity grows and strengthens, the way in which we behave can also alter, further increasing the positivity in our minds and lives. Positive affirmations are most effective when used alongside some other techniques and strategies recommended to aid in combatting impostor syndrome, such as visualisation.

Affirmations can be useful prior to high stress situations, for example if you are about to give a presentation in front of a group of clients or colleagues. They can provide a focus on positivity and repeating affirmations acknowledging your knowledge, experience, skills, and competence to complete the task ahead. This will have the effect of creating a sensation of calm and confidence, and put your mindset in a good place to succeed at your task.

Examples of positive affirmations include:

• I have the tools I need to succeed at my job.

• I am good enough.

• I have the skills I need to succeed at my job.

• I am worthy.

• I am confident in my abilities.

• I will speak with confidence.

• I acknowledge my self-worth.

• I choose not to take constructive criticism personally.

• My opinion matters.

• I know what I am doing.

• It is ok to make mistakes. I will learn and grow from them.

• I am improving and growing constantly.

• I am calm and I control my emotions.

• I move past stress to calm.

• Challenges are opportunities to grow and progress.

• I am intelligent and talented.

• I let go of fearing failures and mistakes.

• Feelings are not facts.

• I am calm and confident.

• I will not compare myself to others.

Affirmations can aid in improving low self-esteem, and have been used to aid the treatment of those with some mental health conditions, including anxiety and depression. The way positive affirmations work and affect the pathways in the human brain stimulates the brain's regions that improve the likelihood of us affecting real positive change that can benefit our physical and mental health. If we feel good about ourselves, with healthy levels of self-esteem and self-worth, we are far more likely to behave in ways to improve our own well-being.

By using positive affirmations, we can improve self-esteem and confidence, improve productivity and improve our ability to keep the negative feelings under control, including the likes of anger, frustration, and impatience, which can all be disruptive and destructive emotions. Affirmations can also be helpful in the setting of personal goals as, once the goal is defined, positive affirmations can be designed specifically to help keep you motivated and moving onwards towards success.

What gives affirmations their effectiveness is frequent repetition. To be truly effective, these repetitions need to start at the first signs of the negative behaviours and thoughts that are causing problems.

To create positive affirmations designed to work for your particular areas of negativity, set some quiet time when you can think about the situations that you want to change. Note down the behaviours and automatic thoughts that you want to change. If this feels overwhelming to begin with, try to stay calm and remember that, even though feelings are definitely important, feelings are not facts. The negative thoughts that plague your life make life very difficult, but they are not the truth of you. Your impostor syndrome might be telling you that you are under-qualified or not good enough, but the objective facts state the opposite. Use the facts to create affirmations that will corral those thoughts and help you to feel the truth of the situation much more accurately.

It is important to create and frame the affirmations in a way that gives the most motivation to keep going and working to achieve them successfully. To do this, make sure that they are created from the genuine facts of the situation and are realistic and achievable. Do not fall into the trap of trying to project a false image unsupported by the objective facts, as this is a central element of impostor syndrome and will make the situation worse rather than better. Make sure also that what you need to say, do, or think, fits in with your moral values and view, so that the risk of making the problem even worse is reduced.

Look at the specific negative thoughts identified as correlating with the situations and interfering with your confidence in them. Identify the statements that the negative thoughts are feeding into your mind. This enables the selection of a statement as a positive affirmation specifically designed to counteract that specific negative thought and convert it to a positive one. 'I am capable of doing this, because I have the qualifications and experience' would be an example of a targeted affirmation to counter a specific negative thought of being underqualified to handle a task.

Some people find affirmations to be more effective if written in the present tense, so that the statement is framed as something that is happening right now, like 'I am worthy,' for example. Others find that future tense works perfectly well for them, as in 'I will grow in experience and knowledge every day,' so it is really a case of seeing what works best for you, whether you need the statement framed as being true in the moment, or as something that will come to pass.

Say it as if you mean it. The more emotional weight you put in to the affirmation, the more effective it is likely to be. Really meaning it when you say it shows that you really do want this thing to happen. Make the affirmation important to you, and project that importance and meaning into the saying of it, or thinking of it if you do not feel confident enough to speak your affirmations aloud to yourself yet.

Remember that this is a procedure, a series of steps that needs to be followed over time. Remember not to put pressure on yourself to fix the negative thoughts overnight. The likelihood is that these thoughts and behaviours did not appear and become the habitual problem they have become overnight. This is working to alter patterns of thinking and behaviour that have in all probability fallen into place over years of being practiced. Neural pathways in the brain can be changed, but it takes time. Combatting impostor syndrome is not a quick process. It takes determination and perseverance. The hard work is worth the effort when the power and hold of the negative thoughts on your brain begins to loosen, and you can begin to acknowledge and appreciate your worth and value as a person and as a professional.

Once you have your positive affirmations structured to help you counter the negative automatic thoughts and lessen their impact and influence on your professional life, you can continue with the process of cognitive restructuring. While some of the steps detailed here are similar to those raised earlier, they are all included here to enable smooth following of the process involved in cognitive restructuring.

## Talk it out

As with other approaches, finding and talking to trusted people can really help. Finding that you are not alone in these feelings and doubts cuts down the sense of isolation impostor syndrome can instil. Trusted peers, particularly those with as much or more experience than you that you respect can demonstrate just how those fears and doubts are unfounded, reassuring you that you are competent and good at what you do and providing a sense of mental peace as your self-esteem and self-confidence raises.

## Understand areas of strength and weakness

Having areas of your life, knowledge, or skillset

that could use some work to improve does not mean that you are a failure and no good at what you do. We are all works in progress, and all have different areas of strength and weakness. Take time to think about it and make lists of each. When you have these lists, they can be used as a reality check when you are doubting yourself in an area listed as a strength, and give you a resource to see what you can do to improve areas defined as weaker. It may be that, with a bit of thinking and focus, you may be able streamline your services to avoid any particularly weak areas being a problem if improving them would be difficult.

## Remember nobody is perfect

Linked in part to the previous paragraph and remembering that nobody is capable of doing everything perfectly, make sure that the goals you set yourself for your performance and career are realistic and achievable, while making them suitably challenging to keep your career and experience progressing. When mistakes happen, as they do for everybody sometimes, learn not to see them as a reason for shame, but as an opportunity to learn how to do things better next time.

## Create a quick response strategy

While the aim is to conquer impostor syndrome and remove its ability to interfere with your life, the process of combatting its power to influence you is not speedy. While working on the overall problem, it is very useful to have a plan in place to deal with impostor syndrome at moments of stress from early in the process.

An effective way to achieve this is to create some separation between yourself and the power the negative thoughts can inflict emotionally. Thinking about situations in the third person rather than the first person makes them much less personal, and can remove some of the sting of embarrassment if something has not gone quite to plan, or take away a little of the trepidation when planning how to handle an upcoming situation. Instead of 'Why did I...' use the phrasing 'Why did they...' and there will instantly be a more objective feeling to the thoughts as the perspective moves to the external.

Although it seems intimidating and counter-intuitive, one way to halt the feeling of being inadequate and not taking enough risks is to increase the amount of risks you take. It sounds strange to contemplate, risking more to counter a fear of risk and being found wanting, but taking carefully selected risks can pay off in increased confidence. Taking carefully calculated risks and completing them successfully can make a powerful statement to counteract your critical inner voice, although it is important to select the risks with care, and avoid the temptation to be reckless, as recklessness can backfire and lead to self-sabotage.

## Allow yourself to accept your successes

It is often very difficult for those with impostor syndrome to accept positive feedback and compliments, and to believe in their truth. Instead, they will come up with 'reasons' why they succeeded, that will 'prove' they do not deserve the praise and accolades coming their way. When things go wrong to any level, on the other hand, they will often accept that without question and blame themselves, sometimes dragging on for far longer than is necessary or good for mental health and well-being. When a task is completed successfully and well, allow yourself to understand the truth of your part in that. Also remember that the person giving the positive feedback and praise is likely to be well positioned to realise clearly who is responsible for the success. If you have helped a client with a complex dog or they see that their dog is happy and relaxed when they come home after you have walked their dog that day, let yourself see that their perspective, their view of the situation is valid. Learn to absorb and accept that. If they are telling you good things that they feel about what you have done for them, listen to them. If your client is happy with you, there is a good reason for that, and it is not any excuse. It is because you have done what they asked of you, and they can see that. You may not be able to see it in the beginning, but with time and practice at accepting that praise, you will begin to see it as well.

# COGNITIVE BEHAVIOURAL THERAPY

Cognitive Behavioural Therapy (CBT) is a scientifically developed and evaluated type of therapy, which focuses on how we think, feel, and behave to help us understand and deal with emotional and behavioural problems. This particular form of therapy is rapidly growing in popularity. This is largely because of the effectiveness and efficiency with which it works for a range of different psychological problems. There are professional CBT qualified therapists available, and for those dealing with severe issues, it is strongly recommended that they seek help from a suitably qualified and experienced professional. For less serious problems, with some basic techniques, it is very possible for many to become their own therapists.

One of the things that makes CBT so effective, especially for a problem like impostor syndrome, is the educational aspect of this form of therapy. The practical approach of CBT educates people in how to look at their thought processes, immediate emotional reactions, and behaviours. It then instructs in how to identify the ones that are not helpful, or are harmful, and how to develop effective, healthy strategies to deal with them. This educational approach is most likely responsible for the fact that studies have revealed CBT to be more effective in the long term, with fewer cases seen to relapse, than other forms of psychotherapy used for similar problems, or the use of medication alone. This has been seen in research, including for anxiety and depression, both of which conditions bear close links with impostor syndrome as mentioned earlier in the book.

The essential basis of CBT techniques may seem like they should be considered as basic common sense and sensible practical approaches to the problem. One of the central characteristics of being human is that, particularly in situations we find stressful or distressing, common sense can go out of the window, and the simplest concepts can seem almost impossible to complete. CBT is not a fast solution to the problem, but with some time and effort, it makes it possible to avoid the mental flapping and panic that interfere with good sense type thinking.

So what does Cognitive Behavioural Therapy mean?

These are the individual word definitions as found on dictionary.com:

Cognitive:
1: of or relating to cognition; concerned with the act or process of knowing, perceiving, etc.: cognitive development; cognitive functioning.
2: of or relating to the mental processes of perception, memory, judgment, and reasoning, as contrasted with emotional and volitional processes.

Behavioural:
1: manner of behaving or acting.
2: Often behaviours, a behaviour pattern.

Therapy:
1: the treatment of disease or disorders, as by some remedial, rehabilitating, or curative process:
2: a curative power or quality.
3: any act, hobby, task, program, etc., that relieves tension.

To add some slightly less formal and more friendly definitions, cognitive involves all of our mental processes, including thinking, dreams, memories, our attention span, and mental images. Behaviour is the things we do, including how we act, what we say and any way in which we might avoid doing things. A therapy is a systematic method of dealing with a problem, mental or physical condition, or illness.

To work from these definitions, therefore, CBT involves the processes of how we think and act. Further to this, it works by assessing how we think and behave and altering the thought and behaviour patterns that harm our well-being. CBT then involves replacing them with other healthier and more constructive thoughts and acts, to provide a method of treatment to reduce as far as possible the unhelpful, harmful thinking and behaviour patterns. Because of the way that CBT states our thoughts, behaviours and emotions link together, using the principle that the way you think is the way you feel, if your thoughts are productive, happy, and rational, your life is more likely to be happy and productive also.

CBT is a scientific approach. There is a lot of scientific research and studies backing up the use of CBT, meaning that this therapy has been well tested and developed scientifically. It also appeals to many people due to its method of teaching people to be scientific themselves in the way they examine their own thoughts and behaviours.

CBT combines this scientific approach with a philosophical element. All humans are individuals, with a unique combination of thoughts and feelings, beliefs and values that make up their core personalities and mindset. These beliefs and values concern themselves, other people, and the entirety of the world around them. One function that CBT is designed to attempt is to aid people in developing beliefs that are helpful rather than harmful, not extreme and are flexible. Flexible beliefs are important, as they are more readily adapted to take into account reality. When we consider the issue of impostor syndrome, reality is a central concept of which we must be aware. While one of the main principles of CBT is that changing how we think and act is a large part of what we need to do to effect real change and development, it realises that thoughts and acts are not the whole picture. We can work on changing what goes through our minds, the emotions that we feel, and what we do in consequence of those things, but there are also elements that we cannot completely alter. Although we can choose the environments in which we immerse ourselves to an extent, we cannot always completely change them, and the environments in which we surround ourselves can have major effects on our ways of thinking and mindset. Our environments contain factors that we can have no control over, including things such as other people and the dynamics in the workplace among others. For this reason, the ability to be flexible in what we believe is a vital one for us to live comfortably in our own minds. Nobody can be in control of everything around them, but they themselves are something over which they can exercise influence in any environment, so working to alter the negative and disruptive patterns of their thinking and behaviour can make changes in the way they feel, without requiring any change in the situation around them.

CBT also puts a focus on actions that we can take to change thinking patterns, emotional reactions, and the behaviours that are associated with stressful, difficult situations. When mired in the depths of impostor syndrome, it can feel as if getting out of it is all but impossible. CBT is a structured therapy, one that focuses on taking action. The very act of doing something about a problem can be helpful in its own right, and provide further motivation to keep going and working at improving things. CBT helps with that, as it makes available a range of techniques that build into a virtual toolkit allowing you to work through the process from the reactive problematic thinking and actions towards what you define as the goals you would feel more comfortable with as your established thought and behaviour patterns. CBT is logical and methodical, moving from step to step and solving problems in a progressive manner.

## How does Cognitive Behavioural Therapy work?

As mentioned earlier, CBT has developed through an extensive process of scientific evaluation, meaning that it is a proven method of helping manage and combat a number of psychological problems. CBT functions from the position of challenging how we think about things and thinking them through in detail, then trying new things and strategies for dealing with situations. By the processes it uses to analyse thoughts and feelings, and the behaviours that result from them, CBT demonstrates that some of the habits and strategies developed up until this point to aid in coping with emotional problems can actually keep the problems ongoing or even make them worse.

As CBT is very much driven by the individual receiving the therapy and their specific thoughts and emotional responses, it is a highly personalised form of therapy. It focuses in on precisely how the person views things, their thoughts and feelings, and the personal interpretations and meanings they attach to events when determining their emotional responses to situations.

CBT does not actually focus on finding a 'root cause' for problems, although the therapy structure can aid in dealing with issues from the past if those historic events have an effect on the current problems and the associated thoughts and emotions. If looking at history can help with current reactions and feelings, CBT can certainly consider those past occurrences. Other than for this purpose, finding the cause is not really pursued to any depth, in favour of a greater focus on examining how thoughts, emotions, and behaviours maintain the problems and are unhelpful, possibly even harmful.

The central way in which CBT functions to help problems like impostor syndrome and other common types of emotional issues is by providing practical steps and methods to follow in developing management strategies. These strategies develop into a kind of psychological toolkit to help control and overcome the effects of impostor syndrome and associated anxiety problems, among others. The educational element is a large part of what makes CBT so effective, more so in the long term than a number of different alternatives. By teaching proven techniques, CBT enables the impostor syndrome sufferer to be their own therapist, certainly on a day-to-day basis. This means that the therapy can be undertaken any time it is needed to challenge negative thought and behaviour patterns, and find better ways to deal with situations that result in negative emotions and those unhelpful and unhealthy thinking and behavioural patterns.

CBT does not claim it will find the 'hidden source' of your problems but rather strives to change unhelpful or harmful thinking and behavioural rituals and emotional responses to more 'normal' and less emotionally distressing ones. CBT will also take into account the fact that the reality of having an emotional problem can prompt further emotional problems to compound the issues. Common examples would be feeling embarrassment or shame at the fact of being anxious or depressed.

One of the pillars on which CBT is based is the way in which an individual person's interpretation of the world and the beliefs they hold about themselves, others, and the world around them affect their perceived experiences and interactions with those people and things. This goes back to the central idea that 'you think how you feel' so that a person that is feeling bad, in an unhelpful pessimistic or anxious way, is very likely thinking in a bad or unhelpful way. This is usually not a deliberate act on their part, and they may well not actively realise that they are feeling that way, but that final result is still the same.

## Connecting feelings, thoughts, and behaviour

Taking into consideration the connection between the way a person thinks and feels and their behaviour, one of the tools that CBT utilises early in the process to help gain perspective on thoughts and emotional responses is what is known as the ABC formula. This formula can be worked through every time negative thoughts and emotions arise in what appears to be a response to something in particular. Negative feelings linked with impostor syndrome can include the following and more: fear, shame, embarrassment, anxiety, guilt around the concept of success, lack of self-worth, low self-confidence, and depression.

Once the negative emotion has been identified, designate that as 'C'. In CBT, this may often be referred to as the emotional and behavioural consequence.

The next step is to look for what started that particular feeling off, whether that is a particular situation or an internal thought. This trigger receives the title 'A'. As it is the thing that starts the negative thinking, it is also known as the actual or activating event.

No matter how it may feel at first, 'A' did not actually cause 'C'. The situation, thought, or whatever occurred just before the negative feeling arrived is not the real cause of the emotional response. In fact, the equation is 'A' + 'B' = 'C'. The final stage in the ABC formula is to identify the 'B', that is the meaning that the individual attaches to the event, their feeling or belief about the trigger 'A' that results in the emotional response that is 'C'.

Once this meaning, belief, or thought is identified, it is then possible to challenge the irrational thoughts that lead the combination of 'A' and 'B' to create 'C'. When the challenge to the irrational thinking has taken place and shifted the thoughts and beliefs about the situation or event to a more rational form, the effect and influence of the negative thoughts reduces. In time, it may be possible to reduce completely the negative thoughts linked with that trigger. In this way the trigger becomes more of a neutral stimulus. It may still be a situation that is not welcomed, but can be accepted and lived with, without having a negative effect on mindset or outcome.

To put it in simpler terms, the meanings and feelings attached to an event have an effect on the emotional responses that event provokes in the individual. Positive associations prompt positive responses such as joy, excitement, or happiness. Negative associations promote negative emotional responses, including anxiety or sadness. These negative associations can play into the experience of impostor syndrome, and cause the sufferer to extrapolate suppositions and meanings from their emotional responses that may have no basis in fact and reality. These inaccurate conclusions can lead to the meanings attached to some events being extreme, with the potential to cause a lot of mental and emotional disturbance and distress.

Say for example that someone has applied for a new job, but does not get the post. This may have them feeling down and bad. The ABC formula for this situation could flow as follows:

A: The potential employer does not give the job to this person (the event).
B: The unsuccessful applicant may start to experience thoughts such as 'I'm no good at this job and I never will be!' (the meaning/belief).

C: The unsuccessful applicant feels bad as they feel themselves to be incompetent, lacking in talent or ability (the emotional consequence).

There is nothing really wrong with feeling a little sad and possibly frustrated for a while over not getting hired if the job is a really wanted one. It becomes unhealthy when this feeling is not temporary but persists and possibly intensifies with dwelling on it, and the sufferer develops the extreme view that not being hired on this one occasion means they are no good at the job and will never manage to make any progression in their career. Extreme conclusions based on a very small number of occurrences and using them to relate to the world at large, all the situations that can arise and people that can be encountered, is very unhelpful and can move a mindset from distressed to disturbed.

The APA Dictionary of Psychology has the following definition of emotional disturbance:

a fear-, anxiety-, or other emotionally based condition that results in maladaptive behaviour—ranging from withdrawal and isolation to acting out and aggression—and adversely affects an individual's academic and social functioning.

To put it more simply, the term 'disturbed' when used by psychologists refers to the type of emotional responses that are not helpful and can be very uncomfortable and potentially harmful. Specifically in CBT, 'disturbed' refers to the way these responses and the behaviour patterns that can follow perpetuate the cycle of negative thinking around the perceived troublesome events. CBT helps identify these meanings, these thoughts and beliefs that come with emotional disturbance, and provides tools to substitute those extreme thoughts with others that are not as extreme and bear much closer resemblance to the real facts of the situation. This can then lead to the corresponding reduction in extremity of the resulting emotional and behavioural consequences.

In the case of our unsuccessful job seeker, the assumed meaning of 'I'm no good at this' can, with rational thought applied, be converted to 'I didn't really click with the interviewer,' or possibly 'The other candidate may be a little more experienced than me, so it might be better next time,' for example. The emotional response then might be a period of disappointment which will pass, and be a much healthier mental state than persistently feeling bad and thinking that you will never get the job you want.

How then to identify whether the beliefs and meaning attached to events are accurate and rational, or whether they are irrational and negative and with the potential for causing emotional disturbance? Some targeted questions can challenge the thinking, and allow perspective on whether it is fuelling negative emotional responses and impostor syndrome. If the answers are mostly in the affirmative, then it is likely that the thinking is flawed and leading to what is actually unnecessary emotional disturbance.

Is this meaning biased against you?

Does it make you feel worse about yourself?

Does it make you feel like giving up?

Will it lead you to stop striving towards your end goal?

Are your thoughts around this event more extreme than they should be?

Are you giving this event and your thoughts surrounding it far too much power over you and your life?

Are the conclusions that you take from it more harsh and all defining than they should be, whether about yourself, others, or the entire world around you?

Are you permitting a single event or small number of events to define you in a restrictive fashion?

Are you letting them dictate what the entire path of your life will be?

As mentioned before, CBT considers the links

between how an individual thinks and feels, and the way they act or behave. With that in mind, there are behaviours that also need watching out for, as they can make the situation worse. Anxiety can cause avoidance of situations perceived to be dangerous or threatening, and avoidance further increases anxious feelings about the situation, compounding the issue. By avoiding a situation, the opportunity to combat the fear and overcome the issue will never arise, and things will never really improve. Depression can lead to withdrawal and increasing isolation. Isolation type behaviours like not seeing other people will lower the mood further and make that feeling even worse. Some can be harmful physically as well as mentally. Using alcohol or drugs as a crutch for mental discomfort can easily become self-destructive and dangerous.

## Problematic thinking

CBT sometimes refers to problematic thinking as 'thinking errors', glitches in thought patterns that we can all make sometimes, and that interfere with the ability to accurately and realistically assess your talents, skills, abilities, and experience level.

This lack of accuracy can result in faulty conclusions. This is, of course, fertile ground for the mentally draining impostor syndrome and its tendency to make sufferers think the worst of themselves professionally and personally. With some help regarding knowing what to look out for and how to identify and isolate the flawed thinking, the ability develops to create some distance and remove the personal sting. This makes challenging the thinking easier.

These potential problems thought patterns could trip the mind and push the sufferer to doubt their own abilities and talents. Here we will look at some of these thought patterns and how to challenge them.

## No, you are probably not clairvoyant

The way in which impostor syndrome makes sufferers doubt themselves means that new tasks and projects are likely to start with an expectation of failure. When mentally predicting the path of events, problematic thinking might only permit anticipating a negative outcome, when the reality is that failure may well not be the most probable result.

Rather than trying to predict the future, it is much healthier to see the situation through with no negative expectations. Discover the result when it happens, untainted by pessimism and negativity. Spend enough time thinking that things will not work out, and there comes a risk of avoiding trying things, or that the repeated prophecies of failure become self-fulfilling.

Calculated risks, trying something that rational analysis shows has a very good chance of success, can help to challenge impostor syndrome thinking. In many cases, the more a sufferer can see the impostor thoughts disproved, the less influence the impostor thinking will be able to have on them. A little risk, when the negative thoughts are more controlled, can also make life much more interesting.

Embrace the concept of trying to do something despite the feelings of trepidation. The impostor feelings are not the truth of the matter. Push through them and see what happens. When what happens is success, those predictions lose some of their power. If they did not come true this time, why should they next time?

As stated previously, mistakes happen. Things can sometimes go wrong or shift out of your control. These things happen to all of us at some time or another. The fact that they have happened once does not mean that they will happen again. This demonstrates the importance of learning to forgive yourself for any mistakes or misjudgements and seeing them as learning opportunities, accepting that sometimes things happen without being your fault. Dwelling on them and beating yourself up mentally for them will never result in a positive mental outcome. Absorb any lessons, allow yourself to feel disappointment or sadness for a short time, but move on before the feelings linger for an inappropriate time and drag you down.

# One blip does not equal disaster

This is sometimes known as an 'all-or-nothing' mindset, or 'black-or-white' thinking, meaning that a situation is expected to result in one of two extreme outcomes. This kind of thinking means an expectation that situations will end in either complete success or total failure. It bears strong links to the perfectionist tendencies known to be prevalent in many cases of impostor syndrome.

These extremes of thinking—perfection or disaster, success or failure, it's all my fault or it's nothing to do with me—can lead to extremes of behaviour. It is also highly possible that, when any kind of failure is interpreted as complete disaster, any setback at all can result in a new project or task being given up, abandoned without a fair chance of completion. The human brain allows this type of thinking to have power quite easily, proclaiming that only perfection will do and anything less is worthless.

To counter this kind of thinking requires learning to think not in strictly black or white but instead in shades of grey. Life is not a string of absolutes, of rights and wrongs, but of degrees, somewhere in the middle. Difficult as it may seem to be when locked into that all-or-nothing mindset, failure and success can co-exist. Failing one element of something does not mean the entire process should be abandoned. It is possible to fail at something and learn from it, pick yourself up and try again, and succeed, despite the earlier setback. Nobody can make their way through their life with no mistakes, and to think otherwise is unrealistic and an impossible standard to which to aspire.

The strict restrictive rules dictating the bounds of black-or-white thinking can have severe effects on the ability to try new things and stretch boundaries, in case something goes wrong and throws the whole idea into jeopardy. It is far better to realise that life is measured in degrees, and to realise that it goes on after a mistake. Flexibility of expectations can only be a good thing.

# Build resilience and pliability into your thinking

Connected with the idea of getting stuck in black-or-white thinking is the difficulty surrounding inflexibility in thinking. Resilience in thinking is a much better way to exist.

According to dictionary.com resilience is defined as:

1: the power or ability to return to the original form, position, etc., after being bent, compressed, or stretched; elasticity.
2: ability to recover readily from illness, depression, adversity, or the like; buoyancy.

Resilience and flexibility of thinking is a great thing to promote for anybody, but for those with a tendency to become locked in to harmful thought patterns it is particularly beneficial. Inflexible thinking does not allow the mind to adapt and mould according to the reality of the situation, and keeps it locked into beliefs that may not be accurate or valid. Below are some examples of thoughts that can be unhelpful.

*Everyone should have the same ideals and stick to them.* While in some ways it would be wonderful if we all lived by the same ideals and with the same priorities, we do not. We can only be responsible for ourselves. Others will have their own priorities, and their own way of doing things, and that is absolutely fine. Accept that fact and remove that stress from yourself.

*Needing validation from others.* This is a common problem for those with impostor syndrome. Thinking that approval from others is an essential can cause a lot of mental distress if that approval is not forthcoming. A far healthier outlook is to allow that a preference for external validation is fine, but to regard it as a need is not healthy. It is better by far to find ways to replace it with internal validation, accepting and absorbing your own ability to realise your self-worth.

*Fixating on the idea of how things 'should' be.* While having ideas on the ways of doing things is fine, letting those rigid ideas dictate your mental state in any way is not. Other people may have different standards according to which they live. While you can control your own standards, ideas and behaviour, you cannot have control over others. Flexibility and resilience in thinking can allow you to be accepting of that fact. Live by those standards as your life allows, but do not be too rigid about how everything 'has' to be. Leave a little wriggle room to accept that things do not always go quite to plan, and that others may have different ideals and standards by which they live. The other person may not do things the way you believe they 'should' but, as long as there is no moral objection to how they are doing things, let them do their own thing their own way, and find ways to work together.

*Not remembering to look out for your own welfare.* It is very easy to become fixated on the idea of 'letting other people down' which can feed into the workaholic tendencies typical to many with impostor syndrome. Another potential cause for not looking after yourself sufficiently is lacking the confidence to assert yourself in situations, meaning as a result ending up doing more than a fair share of the work. This leads into developing feelings of stress and anxiety that can, if not addressed, result in severe anxiety and/or depression.

## Facts, not feelings

Our feelings and emotions are powerful but

letting them dictate matters is a mistake, as feelings can be fallible. This is particularly true for those with impostor syndrome. Allowing your feelings to lead you can result in vanishing down a never-ending rabbit hole, chasing the cause for those feelings. Waking up in the morning with a sense of worry with no identifiable cause for instance can prompt an obsession with working out what 'must' be wrong for you to feel that way.

Our subconscious minds do not work in a clear way that seems logical to the conscious mind, therefore it is possible for the subconscious to introduce some vague, ill-defined feeling of dread that serves no real purpose, but which puts your mind on alert, looking for the cause. Equally, the thoughts could be fragments left from a dream, forgotten on waking, that has no truth in the light of day but it persists. It is worth noting that these feelings can also be signs of psychological disturbances or disorders such as anxiety or depression, which would need to be resolved to aid in recovering the best mental balance that you can. Professional help should be sought if severe psychological symptoms are present.

When it seems as if emotions are overtaking facts, it is worth examining the resulting thoughts to attempt regaining control of the runaway feelings. Identify the emotions involved, and what those emotions are pushing you to conclude, and remind yourself of the difference between feeling and fact, between emotion and the reality of the situation. Do not accept your first feelings about a situation without question, as you cannot always rely upon them as valid.

If, on closer examination, there is no obvious and rational cause for the feeling, push past it. Do not let poorly defined and baseless fears stop you from doing something 'just in case' a vague sense of unease is trying to unsettle you. Think about how you would feel in this situation if not feeling worried and stressed. Are your feelings forcing you to draw false conclusions not based in facts? Is there any rational reason to think that a bad thing is coming?

When you do find yourself in the grip of an emotional response, do not expect that reaction to disappear immediately, even if you find evidence that the feeling is baseless. Emotions prompt physiological changes in the body, some of which are described in the earlier section on stress and the fear response, and the effects of these changes will not dissipate in an instant. Give the feelings time to subside, and then it will be possible to look back at those feelings and perhaps gain an insight into where they come from. Remember that it does not necessarily have to be an event that prompts these feelings to arrive. Emotional responses including unspecified anxiety or worry can be due to extreme tiredness or as a hangover from a previous emotional state.

# Rejecting Recognition

This links to the impostor syndrome tendency to discount approval and praise, deflecting it by attributing any success to external factors. Luck, being in the 'right place at the right time', or thinking what has been achieved is simply not that difficult because you have managed it are all thoughts that connect to the inability to perceive the positives in your own performance. They all leach out the positive effects the result actually has, leaving the impostor syndrome sufferer with at best a neutral feeling, but quite possibly a lingering sense of negativity connected to the event.

To combat this tendency, the ability to take compliments with grace and belief in their truth and validity may require some practice. Remember that the speaker's opinion on what has happened is valid. If a client decides that you have really helped them and their dog, then it is their truth. Is it not really their decision whether or not you have helped them? Take note of what they say, your good points that they have brought up. With time, you can come to realise that their words hold the truth. The more you can manage to accept compliments, the easier it will become.

## Twisting the truth

A mental filter is a distortion held in the mind

that twists the facts to fit an existing mindset. It only allows for acceptance of those facts that fit with an existing belief. Anything that does not correspond with that belief is discounted or ignored, regardless of the truth of the situation. Those achievements and positives exist, whether you can see them or not. Remembering that fact may help when it comes to battling that mental filtering process.

To fight against this mental filtering, a helpful tool is to gather evidence that directly goes against these erroneous negative beliefs and disproves them, to bring the negative bias back towards truth. Objective, fact-based evidence that is verifiable, such as qualifications in your area of work are excellent examples. There is no subjective interpretation of a qualification gained. This means that your mental filter cannot deny the truth of it. As the filter loses its strength, positive feedback and praise can be included more as you learn to accept it and not discount its value.

Also examine how your thought patterns differ when looking at somebody else's career. In all likelihood, you will be much more accepting of their abilities and less prone to writing them off as not corresponding to a belief. Try to view your own accomplishments and achievements with the same fairness and openness. Otherwise the negative bias and filtering will continue and be compounded.

# Leave the labels

At first glance, labels seem little more than convenient identifiers of things, and they are all around us. In many cases, however, labelling can be extremely restrictive. To apply a label to an inanimate object is one thing, but to label a living being is a poor idea. Living things are in a constant state of change, and cannot be reduced to one or two words that cannot possibly accurately encompass their complex natures.

Labelling of oneself can be harmful to mental balance. If you label yourself in a negative way, such as 'bad' or 'incompetent' it will have continuing negative effects on your thoughts, dragging them down further. Labelling yourself in some way that denotes poor abilities or failure is also extremely self-limiting, as it does not take into account that mistakes can happen and things go wrong outside of your control. Examples of labels that should definitely be avoided include phrases such as 'I'm incompetent', 'I'm a failure', 'I'm not good enough' and similar.

Resist the urge to apply labels, and concentrate instead on accepting the facts at face value, without the restrictions of labels that cannot possibly take into account the whole truth of you or your situation.

# Avoid avoidance

Although avoidance behaviours can seem like a good idea at the time (if a situation makes you anxious or worried, staying away must be better, right?) it can be very restrictive or harmful in the long term. Avoiding situations entirely removes the opportunity to work on that fear and anxiety, and removes the chance to work on testing and stretching yourself. The more situations you permit yourself to avoid and do not attempt to face, the more it could become a default choice, further restricting your life. It may provide a measure of relief from stress in the short term by staying away from the worrying thing, but increases it in the long term, having more and more effect on your life as it builds to a larger mental block. Avoidance is an example of a behaviour that can maintain or actually make a problem like impostor syndrome worse.

As well as avoiding situations altogether, another form of avoidance is to wait until being in the 'right frame of mind'. This is a form of procrastination, and common in impostor syndrome. The issues with waiting are that it can leave a mountain to do to complete a task, or that the 'right' time and 'right' mood will never come.

# Generalising is generally a bad idea

There can be a tendency for us as human beings to leap to conclusions quickly. Included in this is the idea of deciding things about ourselves, others, or events, based on very few or even a single factor or occurrence.

This can be extremely damaging. Forming an opinion of our intelligence or competence in the moments after experiencing a failure or something going wrong will result in erroneous and upsetting conclusions.

Perspective is vital when it comes to assessing the impact of things going wrong. Before being tempted to conclude that you cannot do anything right professionally, for example, take a moment to assess the reality of that thought. Do things truly always go badly for you? Do you truly never get things right professionally? When viewed without the negative filter in place, the truth of the matter can be seen, and will be much more balanced than the generalisation allows for.

When things do go wrong, or mistakes are made, do not draw conclusions but instead make a note of what can be done differently or better next time, as this is far more constructive and kinder on yourself, and your mental balance and well-being.

# SELF-ESTEEM AND SELF-ACCEPTANCE

Self-esteem is a concept strongly connected to self-worth and the impostor syndrome type of thinking. Low self-esteem often shows in tendencies towards negative emotions, such as anxiety, shame, guilt, etc. If these are frequent experiences, then low self-esteem could well be an issue.

It is a perhaps sad fact that, in this modern world, there is a constant pressure to be 'the best' at something. It is no longer enough for many to be very able at a particular thing, unless there is some method of proving to be better than others around us. This has created a strong tendency to arise to be highly achievement driven. Not only driven by these achievements but basing self-worth and self-esteem on them, and possibly them alone. The problem with viewing our worth only in terms of such temporary measures of success is that if something goes astray, such as not passing an assessment for example, it means our self-worth and self-esteem can all but disappear as a result. Far better to find other measures by which to calculate your own sense of worth, and realise that it is far more important who you are than what others have seen you do.

Rather than basing your opinion of yourself on external factors, it is far more constructive and healthy to work from a position of self-acceptance. If you can accept yourself as you are, and base your self-esteem and self-worth on that foundation of self-acceptance, it is far less likely to go down, cause mental distress, and lead further down the path towards impostor syndrome.

Self-acceptance removes the potential for lowering self-esteem as it does not depend on rating yourself, but instead on being able to accept yourself as you are. When you are working from a basis of self-acceptance, you see your own worth as intrinsic, belonging naturally.

Self-acceptance means realising a number of things about human beings and humanity. Humans are complex and individual; every single one is a unique being. Attempting to place a value on such a unique thing as a human being on some form of set scale is really an impossible task. The fact must also be remembered that, by their very nature, humans are not perfect. We are not robots and so are utterly fallible and capable of making mistakes. As mentioned previously, living things are in a constant state of growth and change, which also makes attributing an arbitrary value of little point.

To begin the process of self-acceptance, you need to first accept that a unique individual cannot be rated against others, because it is not possible to truly compare like with like. There is no value in comparing yourself to others in your family, social, or professional life as none of those people are truly like you enough for a comparison to be anything other than pointless and invalid. Accept that the you of tomorrow will be different to the you of today, who is also different to the you of yesterday. You are ever changing, learning, and growing, Any rating you attach to yourself at one set point will no longer apply, almost from the very moment you assign it.

All beings have worth, as much as any other individual. This includes humans, meaning any person has as much intrinsic worth as any other, regardless of societal conventions that some may see as a definition of worth.

The last item on the list leading towards self-acceptance is the one that many people can find the most difficult. Accepting the fact that as humans we are all fallible and can make mistakes. Being able to accept that fact and forgive ourselves for our mistakes is a massive step towards self-acceptance.

To work towards self-acceptance, we can create a number of beliefs that aid us to accept ourselves as we are. This is not a case of demanding that we believe ourselves to be great from the beginning of the process. These beliefs and attitudes are designed to help forgive the mistakes and errors that we are all bound to make at times. The important things about these beliefs is that they are all logical, realistic, and helpful.

*Logical* refers to the logic of behaviour, and the gaps between 'must behave this way' and 'prefer to behave this way'. As mentioned before discussing problematic thoughts, preferences in thinking are much easier to live with. Additionally, this flexibility in thinking means that if, for any reason, you cannot act in the preferred manner, preference will allow far more self-forgiveness than rigid thinking, and also takes into account the fallibility of humans, and that we are all capable of making mistakes.

*Realistic* links to the perfectionist tendency that is common to many fighting with impostor syndrome. Perfectionists expect themselves to perform their work perfectly, without fail, every single time. This is not realistic because, as we have already noted, everyone makes mistakes sometimes. A single (or even a few) failures do not destroy all of your hopes and dreams; it is possible to experience failure and go on to succeed. This demonstrates that the urge for perfection is not realistic.

*Helpful* points towards the fact that these beliefs are designed to help self-acceptance. They help move towards appropriate behaviours that are not harmful to mental balance and that allow for appropriate processing of emotions. Rather than aiming to never feel negative emotions (see the previous paragraph about these beliefs being realistic) helpful beliefs allow for negative emotions to be felt and processed for a reasonable amount of time, and then to move on from them.

One of the last things that problematic thinking can push the mind towards, especially for those prone to perfectionism or the inflexible nature of black-and-white thinking, is the belief that to accept something means giving up. When it comes to self-acceptance, this could not be further from the truth. The ability to accept ourselves as we are comes from a position of strength, not weakness. It is something to aim for, not something for which we should feel we have had to settle.

Once these new beliefs and thought patterns are defined, more work is needed to reinforce them in the mind and change the default thinking pathways away from the negative. Telling yourself to believe something is one thing, but actually making the change to truly believing something is another. This, in the initial stages, can lead to a state called cognitive dissonance.

Cognitive dissonance is something that happens when someone holds a belief that goes against another of their beliefs or values, or does something that goes against a belief or value. This clash of beliefs or ideals causes the person to experience a psychological stress response. It causes a mental discomfort, which is a large part of why people may go to great lengths to avoid challenging their thinking. While it may seem easier to avoid the cognitive dissonance, this will not alter the problematic thinking and so the new thinking patterns need reinforcing and practice. While cognitive dissonance is an unpleasant feeling, it is a sign that the troublesome thinking is being challenged, and that the process to improve mental balance has begun.

One way to aid the progress is to behave as if you believe the new way of thinking, even if you are not yet entirely convinced. The term 'fake it until you make it' can be a useful one in these circumstances. The practice of behaving as if you believe will, over time, help cement the new ideas into place. In the beginning, it may be a case of imagining how you might think about things if you did actually believe in this new way, or how people that might hold the same belief would act. As this happens more and more, the new thinking will become the default, and the brain's new neural pathways are set into place.

This is not a quick process, and those old thinking patterns will fight hard to re-establish themselves. One technique to stop them being able to reassert themselves is to prepare some arguments against the old thought patterns that will help in maintaining the new thoughts and beliefs. You can also prepare a list of arguments to support the new thought patterns that you want to promote. These lists of arguments work best for many people written down and kept to read if needed when struggling with the changes in thinking. Depending on how you prefer, this can be on paper or in digital form carried on a device for referral to as and when necessary.

For each of the thoughts, assess them according to the list below:

Is it true or untrue? Working from a position of truth is much easier to maintain and continue.

Is it realistic or unrealistic? Trying to maintain thought patterns and standards that are unrealistic is unfair to yourself, and not sustainable.

Is it logical or illogical? Logical thinking is preferable, as logic is easier to assess with an objective eye.

Is it sensible and sustainable? Trying to change all things at once can be overwhelming. It may be a better idea to work on thinking in stages to avoid becoming flooded and despondent at having overloaded yourself, trying to do too much all at once.

Is it fair and balanced, or is it extreme? Extremes are a bad idea in thinking, as they can lead to drawing radical conclusions from little evidence. Balanced and fair thinking and assessment are preferable to extremes.

Is it flexible or rigid? Rigid thinking is unhelpful, as it does not allow for any variation in situations. Things can change for a variety of reasons with little warning, and flexibility means far more chance of comfortably being able to go with the flow.

Is it helpful or unhelpful? One of the easiest concepts to understand from the outside, but one of the most important in being able to move forwards is the difference in effect of helpful and unhelpful thoughts. Unhelpful thoughts do not permit progression, but hold the mind back in the old, harmful ruts. For tackling unhelpful thoughts, look for helpful alternatives and ways to integrate them into the new, positive, helpful mindset.

# MINDFULNESS

A potentially useful tool to help cut through the noise, particularly in the early stages of combatting impostor syndrome, is mindfulness. This approach aims for a quality of being fully present, observant, and engaged in the current moment. It allows for observing and accepting what is going on at that time while avoiding judgement or distraction, and not becoming caught up in our thoughts or feelings around a situation.

The idea behind mindfulness is to pay deliberate attention to focusing on the present moment, without distractions to interfere with our attention, without allowing the lingering effects of past events or creeping worries about future concerns the moment to unduly influence the moment. The past has been and gone, the future is yet to arrive. This current moment, the one we are in right now, is effectively the only one we have. If we can learn to live in this moment in harmony with all that is going on around us, it can help make our passage through life smoother and less stressful to navigate.

Picture the ocean, with you represented by a boat in the centre of the open expanse of water. All around the boat are waves, echoes of storms in the past or worries about those that might come. Mindfulness aims for calm in the moment, meaning that boat sits on smooth water and, by employing mindfulness techniques, the size of the waves from the past and future effects lessen, as the past and future have less grip on the now. The boat can move on into the quiet waters without worrying about being swamped by the waves. In the same way mindfulness can help prevent the mind becoming overwhelmed by negative thoughts and emotions.

Mindfulness is an ancient practice. The description of the term mindfulness comes from the translations of the Pali word 'sati' meaning 'to remember' and its Sanskrit equivalent 'smrti' which also means 'to remember' as well as 'to bear in mind'. The translations of these words are considered to split into three concepts that sum up the aim of mindfulness.

*Awareness:* if you are not aware of things, they essentially will not exist for you. Without any awareness of the things you have experienced, they have not truly happened for you.

*Attention:* paying attention to the current moment, with complete focus. By practicing mindfulness techniques, you can learn to focus our awareness and attention as you choose, and move it whenever and wherever you wish to.

*Remembering:* mindfulness is about complete immersion in the current moment. This aspect is about remembering to be aware of and pay attention to what you are experiencing in the moment.

Without remembering to focus awareness and attention, human beings tend to live a mindless existence. This means always on the move, bustling from thing to thing, with no real focus on what we are doing right now. It is easy to become distracted and hop back and forth between tasks because there is no focus and real concentration on the task at hand. By employing mindfulness techniques and learning to immerse yourself fully in the moment, you can learn to focus our concentration on a task, enabling effective completion.

## What can mindfulness help with?

Mindfulness can help in managing to relax the body when tense. Tension in the mind when filled with anxious or troublesome thoughts filters through into the body, which will also then tense. This is due to the automatic physical and physiological chain of events that starts as soon as s situation is perceived to be stressful, ready to initiate the fight or flight reactions, as discussed earlier in the book. The body gets itself ready for either running away or fighting for survival. If that energy has nowhere to go, the body tenses up for lack of any other appropriate use of that energy.

Mindfulness can help in learning to manage the patterns of mind and emotions. This means that, with practice, the chance of being overwhelmed by feelings and thoughts is greatly reduced. Negative thought patterns have much less chance of rampaging through our brains and with a resulting plunge into the cycle of despair, lack of self-esteem and mental discomfort all associated with impostor syndrome.

Mindfulness does not actually remove the negative thought or stresses. Instead, mindfulness allows for awareness of those thoughts and feelings that arise in a stressful situation. With that greater awareness comes a heightened ability to choose how to handle those negative thoughts and emotions in the moment. This element of choice gives the chance to separate the thoughts and emotions from the decisions and actions that may need taking in a situation. This means less opportunity for those emotions and restrictive negative thoughts to have an impact on performance and the outcome, and allow them less influence in your life and career.

Mindfulness helps to develop the process of responding to the negative thought patterns and emotions rather than reacting to them. The difference between the two is that a reaction is an automatic knee jerk with no conscious thought attached to the action. A response is a far more considered thing, with the context in which the thoughts and emotions occurred taken into account. This can then permit careful thought and consideration when deciding a path forward. This negates the chance for those harmful automatic thoughts to persist in causing mental distress and damage to future thinking. The sense of distance created and ability to observe thoughts without feeling hurt and saddened so much by them means an ability to analyse them and understand what the reason may be for those particular feelings.

As this ability to accept the less than ideal thoughts but not let them have so much hold over feelings and behaviours develops, the move happens towards not always picturing the worst but instead viewing the world with a more positive, optimistic eye. Taking the time to observe and get to know how your thought patterns evolve and progress through a situation gives the opportunity to develop skills around recognising habits and patterns, and devise methods to avoid them having too much influence. Rather than becoming entangled in the thoughts, it is possible to create some space from the thoughts and emotions, and realise that thoughts are not reality. While it is not possible to control our thoughts, and trying to do so is not a good idea, it is possible to accept that those feelings exist while still acting in a considered way not dictated by those feelings and thoughts.

Removing the negative influence automatically places life into a more positive framework. The effects of stress and anxiety lessen, and the pressures that can come in professional life feel less overwhelming. This will greatly reduce the likelihood of impostor syndrome sinking in its insidious claws and wreaking havoc on your sense of self-worth and self-esteem. The occasional worry about an upcoming new project or task will not go away entirely, but their effects will be far less exaggerated and inappropriate. It is not about stopping the feelings and thoughts altogether, but about not letting them have more power than they rationally should. There is nothing wrong in feeling disappointed or sad if something does not go to plan but, in a well-balanced mind, that feeling disperses and does not linger to keep us feeling bad.

The theory of employing mindfulness is simple but, like any other new skill that you add to your toolbox, it is something that needs practice. The first time that you might sit and try to observe your breathing closely, for example, it is likely that distractions will creep in quickly and break your concentration. It is well worth persevering though as, with that practice put in, the amount of time your concentration span lasts will extend. It may be worth starting out by trying guided meditations if struggling to maintain focus and attention for any length of time in the early stages.

It is estimated that the average person has somewhere between sixty thousand and eighty thousand thoughts per day. With that amazing number of individual things buzzing around in our minds, it is no surprise that they can overwhelm us.

Mindfulness is in fact an innate human ability but can often need some help to come to the fore, especially in our modern, fast paced, technology-filled lives. Mindfulness and meditation are two terms that are often associated together in people's minds. While the two do work in conjunction, mindfulness does not only occur during meditation for those that practice mindfulness as a way of living. Meditation, particularly guided meditation in the first place, is a good way to discover how to become deliberately mindful. When starting out with mindfulness and meditation, the ability to be utterly present in the moment, in the here and now, is gained for a short, limited length of time. With regular practice and regular sessions of mindfulness meditation, you can keep extending those times. With enough consistent practice, the ability can develop to be present in every moment of the day. Using mindfulness techniques allows you to become an observer of your thoughts, able to step back and analyse them without becoming entangled in their ramifications.

One important aspect when in this position of being an observer of your thoughts is to ensure you work from a position of being non-judgemental. This section is talking about mindfulness as a way to rid the mind of the mental distress of impostor syndrome, but the effect is ruined if rather than simply accepting the existence of these thoughts, the fact of having them at all provokes a sense of judgement.

Acceptance is an important point of the process. It is accepting the thoughts and emotions, without judgement as mentioned above, that allows you to be able to move past them. We are all human, we are all fallible, and we are all likely to have thoughts and feelings at times that are not helpful. This feeling of acceptance also extends to situations as well as thoughts. You cannot control everything in the world around us, and trying to do so will only increase stress levels. With acceptance comes the ability to think about how you would choose to respond, rather than the automatic knee jerk reaction that can make you feel worse as a result.

Mindfulness brings benefits in the form of clearing the mind, leading to a state of mental calmness and enabling relaxation. This then leads on to getting better sleep, which further improves all of those things, and permits better concentration on tasks as we choose. You can stay in the moment with that focus and concentration, not caught up in the past or worrying about the future, all of which can help keep impostor syndrome under control. Avoiding mental drama from past events or fear of future occurrences is important, particularly when you may have struggled following past errors or failures that have prompted the gnawing self-doubt of impostor syndrome to take hold. By learning acceptance, it becomes easier to frame those past problems as learning opportunities and inspirations to improve performance in the future.

The danger of letting your mind become bogged down in self-recrimination over past mistakes or things that have gone wrong is self-explanatory, but there is also a huge issue with getting caught up in future worries. By envisaging failure, assumptions are being made, and assumptions are never a great idea. There is some truth to the comedy catchphrase, attributed by some to the American writer Jerry Belson, "Never ASSUME, because when you assume, you make an ASS out of U and ME." When you make assumptions about how situations will work out, you create certain scenarios in our minds, which are not truly connected to reality. Do this often enough and these scenarios begin to feel more and more real with each repetition, and you can create a self-fulfilling prophecy, causing yourself even more problems in the future. This is again where the distance mindfulness can give you from the emotional reactions helps, as you can learn to go with the flow. Rather than anticipating a result, you wait to see how the situation turns out.

Mindfulness can also aid in the process of cognitive restructuring, as discussed earlier in the book. Mindfulness, with its emphasis on observation, allows you to recognise when you are beginning to experience the first feelings of stress. The distance of being an observer of your thoughts and feelings rather than automatically reacting without being able to think means being able to understand why the feelings have arisen. Once you understand that, then you are able to decide rationally how to proceed and lessen the impact of the stress trigger.

Earlier this book looked at the way stress affects the body in the chapter 'Fear of failure and the stress response' earlier in the book. Reducing stress is an important thing to concentrate on, as chronic stress can lead to serious physical and mental health imbalances and illnesses. The text has mentioned the potential connection between the stress of impostor syndrome and the conditions of anxiety and depression, but physical illnesses such as cardiovascular disease and high blood pressure, and unpleasant conditions like Irritable Bowel Syndrome can result if chronic stress is not tackled.

Mindfulness is a healthy way to tackle stress and

reduce its load and effect on the body. As with the CBT approach mentioned previously, writing lists of the things that are causing you stress, the triggers that you identify as starting the stress cycle, and working your way through your list of them tackling each individually is a great way to break the task down into manageable amounts. By working on each individually, you are reducing the chance of becoming overwhelmed by them in bulk, and can tackle them in an order that you are most comfortable with, whether you start with the easiest first, or go for the ones causing most harm to begin with. While you cannot completely remove stress from your life, by working through this process and using mindfulness, the effects it has on your life is reduced.

Mindfulness and meditation do not necessarily have to go together, but meditation can be a useful structured way to explore the basic concepts of mindfulness, and help you get the idea of what you are working towards as a result. This is why apps offering guided meditations can be a great place to start if feeling a little confused or struggling to feel that sense of connection with yourself in the moment when first trying mindfulness alone.

The aim of mindfulness meditation is not to empty your mind and think about nothing. Instead, it is designed to direct your focus and attention on a particular thing of your choice, whether internal or external to you. That could be concentrating on your breathing, listening to a piece of music, looking at a picture or a view, as some examples. Breathing or something else connected to the body is often a good choice as it is something familiar, and as it is always with you, it is something you can attempt any time you feel like trying.

Find some quiet time, when you will not be disturbed and have a few minutes guaranteed to be peaceful. Take notice of everything around you, the sights, smells, and sounds in the area you chose for this time. When eating and drinking, do so slowly and savour every mouthful. Really concentrate and taste it. Feel the air moving around your body as you move. Concentrate as you breathe steadily, feeling the sensation of the air moving in and out of your lungs. As you exhale, feel the stress leaving your body along with the breath. This sense of awareness is the essential core of mindfulness. It can be a powerful aid in controlling the effects negative thoughts and feelings of impostor syndrome have on sufferers. The helpful effects of mindfulness are becoming more widely known in aiding the relief of stress and restoring mental balance.

Meditation can be described as either formal or informal in type. Formal meditation means taking set time during the day to meditate deliberately. Meditating with deliberate intent means being able to delve further into your mind, your thoughts and feelings, and understand more how your thought and feeling patterns work and develop. Informal meditation is something that can be done during any point in your day-to-day schedule. When mindfulness and meditation are established as a habit, it becomes much easier to fit them in to your daily life. The more you can do this, the better you can become at it and the greater effect it will have on reducing your stress and enabling you to live a happier life, with much less chance of having your social and professional lives disturbed by the negative thoughts so typical of impostor syndrome.

Some people find the idea of mindfulness difficult to see themselves taking part in. This is often due to misconceptions around what mindfulness is. To those who do not understand, mindfulness may be linked to a kind of spiritualism and somewhat abstract concepts around energy that those who do not follow that kind of thinking find hard to reconcile. If asked what they think of the idea of sitting quietly paying close attention to all that is going on in their immediate environment, they do not react in anywhere near the same way, despite the fact that is a good description of what mindfulness meditation is. Find somewhere quiet where you can be alone, not needing to be concerned about anyone else judging you, and try it, without worrying about what it is called.

There are a number of mindfulness apps available to help develop the ability to be fully present in the moment and aware of your feelings and emotions without letting them control you. There are apps available from free to subscription based. These apps offer guided meditations, often short and designed to follow a daily program to define and develop abilities concerning mindfulness in all areas of life. One of the best known and with many good reviews is Headspace. It is a subscription based service, but offers a free trial period. Contained on the website is a large library of information to help understanding of the subjects of mindfulness and meditation. These links also describe ways in which the techniques can help with a range of matters.

# FINAL THOUGHTS

Impostor syndrome can be a particularly common feeling when we are starting out in a career as some form of canine professional, although one of the nasty tricks it plays on our minds is to make us feel incredibly isolated and alone. For many who feel its effects at some point in their personal and professional lives, it will diminish as their careers grow and develop. For others amongst us maybe a little less confident than those individuals for a wide variety of reasons, it can be far more pervasive and difficult to conquer.

One important thing to remember is that, if you are feeling like an impostor amongst your colleagues and friends, you have clearly reached a certain level of success in your professional world. To feel like an impostor, you must have reached a level to which others would aspire, you are taking those steps on your professional journey. Rock that fact, try to switch the impostor feeling to one of gratitude for the things you must have accomplished to get to this point in your career, and refuse to let any further fear cripple you from climbing higher.

Remember these things when setting out on your journey to combat your impostor syndrome:

You are worthy. Personally and professionally.

You have value, in your life and your profession.

You know more than you admit to yourself right now.

You are more competent and intelligent than you believe yourself to be.

Repeat these to yourself often. They are the truth, and they are a huge part of how you can get past the draining, damaging effects of impostor syndrome.

# ABOUT THE AUTHOR

Jay has been working with and training dogs with more enthusiasm than skill for more years than she cares to remember, largely working Border Collies (or in the case of one very determined dog, NOT working). Although no longer living on the farm or farming sheep, the Border Collie has wormed its way into her heart enough to still be the dog of choice. It was her current dog as he grew and started to struggle with some aspects of life that caused her to begin her research into reactivity and, in the process, discover a new love of learning about dog training and behaviour. A lifelong love affair with the written word has combined with the new interest to inspire her attempt to ensure that no reactive dog owner needs to feel that they are alone.

Other books:

## Fight or Fright? A Reactive Dog Guardian's Handbook

Written by the guardian of a reactive dog and student of canine behaviour, this book sets out to make sure that nobody in that situation has to feel alone. Packed with empathy and understanding, inside is a guide to recognising that your dog is fearful and advice to aid you in finding the help and support that you need to improve life for both you and your reactive dog.

From describing how reactivity impacts on both dog and guardian physically and mentally, to guidance on finding the right kind of professional help, this book will support you on every step of the journey.

## Conversations with Collies

Have you ever looked at the dog at your feet and wondered what life would be like if they could talk?

In the case of my dogs, there would be a lot more sarcasm.

Remembrances from a lifetime of dogs, both of working sheepdog and pet varieties, reconstructed with the input of the dogs themselves. Often amusing, rarely particularly flattering to the people involved.

Maybe it's best to not let them tell us what they're thinking!

Printed in Great Britain
by Amazon